RESTORED BY TRUTH

ASK, BELIEVE IN CHRIST

DONNA KAY ASHLEY PLEASANTS

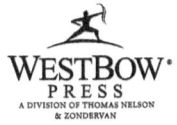

WESTBOW°
PRESS
A DIVISION OF THOMAS NELSON
& ZONDERVAN

Scriptures taken from the Holy Bible, New International Version®, NIV®. Copyright © 1973, 1978, 1984, 2011 by Biblica, Inc.™ Used by permission of Zondervan. All rights reserved worldwide. www.zondervan.com The "NIV" and "New International Version" are trademarks registered in the United States Patent and Trademark Office by Biblica, Inc.™ All rights reserved.

WestBow Press books may be ordered through booksellers or by contacting:

WestBow Press
A Division of Thomas Nelson & Zondervan
1663 Liberty Drive
Bloomington, IN 47403
www.westbowpress.com
1 (866) 928-1240

ISBN: 978-1-4908-3302-6 (sc)
ISBN: 978-1-4908-3304-0 (hc)
ISBN: 978-1-4908-3303-3 (e)

Library of Congress Control Number: 2014906343

Printed in the United States of America.

WestBow Press rev. date: 10/31/2014

I would like to dedicate RESTORED by TRUTH, Ask...Believe...in Christ to my parents, Eunice M. Ashley and Lonzie C. Ashley. God appointed them as my earthly parents and without them I would not be the person I am today. Thank you God!

Also to my beloved son Brooks, to my daughter Shannon and to all the future generations, Restored by Truth, Ask... Believe... in Christ is to be used for their guidance and spiritual training throughout their lives!

*Please note that all scripture references are taken from The New International Version.

*Read the Leader's Guide first, page 127.

CONTENTS

I

FOCAL VERSE ROMANS 12:1-2

Therefore, I urge you, in view of God's mercy, to offer your bodies as living sacrifices, holy and pleasing to God—this is your spiritual act of worship. Do not conform any longer to the pattern of this world, but be transformed by the renewing of your mind. Romans 12:1–2

II

My Testimony

Before we start our process of restoration, I feel the need to share a brief summary of parts of my life for the purpose of connecting and to disarm us of any pride. I do not want you to focus on me, but rather on how God has shown me love and provision.

I would be nothing without Christ. My life would have no direction or purpose. I would not have any peace, nor would I find rest. I would be hopelessly lost in my own personal desert and useless to God. Over the years I have been stuck in my personal deserts. I will be referring to the times and areas of our lives that reflect pain, suffering, addictions, bondage, or sin as personal deserts, the thing or things that we continue to hold on to, even though we know that we should change or let go of them. That something that keeps us stuck in our desert, just as the Israelites were left to wander in the wilderness, or desert, until they became more obedient and willing to earnestly seek God's plan for their lives.

I did not grow up in a strong Christian home with two godly parents, but God provided me with a mother and a grandmother that loved and feared God. My mother, Eunice Marston Ashley, was a strong believer. She taught me about the Bible, she sang the old hymns as she did her work, and she taught me about having an unshakable, childlike faith in Jesus Christ. Without her faith she couldn't have endured what she experienced and still live. She learned all these valuable things from her mother, Marie Marston. My mother revealed her strong faith and belief by calling out to Jesus for help in many times of need throughout her life and many years later on her deathbed. In her final hours she sang the old hymns and conversed with the Lord. I am so blessed to have had a grandmother and a mother that loved me enough to share their faith and love for God with me. I have been thinking about the young man named Timothy about whom the apostle Paul wrote so much. Paul had taken it upon himself to teach Timothy how to be a "man of God." Timothy had a grandmother named Lois, and his mother was named Eunice, for whom my mother was named. Paul's second letter to Timothy reminded Timothy that the origin of his faith came from his grandmother and mother. In 2 Timothy 1:5 Paul wrote, "I have been reminded of your sincere faith, which first lived in your grandmother Lois and in your mother Eunice, I am persuaded, now lives in you also." Now I can write to my children that I have been reminded of their sincere faith, which first lived in their great-grandmother Marie, their grandmother Eunice, and their mother, Donna. I have been blessed beyond measure, God is faithful!

In my early childhood years the Enemy (Satan) attempted to destroy my family by using alcohol to control my dad's life, by making him dependent and out of control. I now understand his dependency upon worldly pleasures, which I believe he used to forget or escape the internalized pain of his upbringing. I am now able to forgive because of seeing him through Jesus' eyes and not my own.

His weekend addiction to alcohol introduced much pain and dysfunction to my childhood. This lifestyle caused all sorts of drama, chaos, and distraction. It lasted into my early twenties, by which time I was married and had a daughter of my own, Shannon. Miraculously, my dad made a complete change in his life; he stopped drinking alcohol and even gave up cigarettes. He became one of the kindest men I have ever known. He has been very kind and generous to my children. I truly believe that he has tried to make up for all the dysfunction in my life, by being such a terrific grandfather. But the damage was already done, and my formative years had passed. I know without any doubt his change came from the constant prayers of my grandmother; she prayed without ceasing. Granny Marston's prayers inspired my mother and me to pray with her for my dad to stop drinking, and for his salvation. By the time I was five, I was taught to pray specifically for my dad. It was a typical weekend to have to flee to Granny's house for refuge, due to all the weekend drama caused by the alcohol abuse. It caused so much pain for my family. The dysfunction was something that I wanted to hide; I wanted to pretend that everything was normal. I learned at a very young age how to disguise my painful feelings, how to hide my anger and to smile when I needed to cry.

I praise God for those weekends at my grandmother's house. I didn't want to leave, because it was the one place that I felt safe and secure. God provided a safe place for me to grow spiritually. I realize now that it was not my grandmother in the flesh that made me feel secure; it was the presence of the Spirit of Christ in her home that gave me a sense of security and stability.

What precious memories I have of being at her house! I was allowed to sleep in my Granny's bed. I can remember her kneeling beside her bed at night. The lights were off, so it was dark in her room, but the moonlight made it possible to see her shadow image, on her knees at her bedside. She would be there for quite a while, praying out loud to God and praising Jesus for all of her blessings. I also remember her sitting in her chair by the fireplace, reading her Bible. She lived a simple life and served her family with joy. She prayed for all her children and grandchildren, and I would hear her call my dad's name too. She always taught me to love and respect my dad regardless of his behavior. She taught me to honor my father because it was one of God's Ten Commandments. She would say, "Don't love the sin, but love the person." She also taught me to pray for my dad and not to ever give up, that with God, all things are possible. I was also taught not to fear but to call out to Jesus when I was in need and afraid. Years later my dad accepted Christ, and he quit using alcohol.

My Granny Marston not only talked about Jesus; she tried to set the example of Him with her simple, uneducated lifestyle. She told me the Jesus stories from the Bible (as a child that is what I called them). I didn't know them as parables or as the "miracles of Jesus," but I heard them all. She knew how to communicate the peace and stability of Christ to a child that felt so abandoned and scared, a child that questioned the outcome of tomorrow. I didn't know then that God was preparing me for the challenges of today. I clearly see how that with each season of my life, God was with me and providing for my each and every need. By spending time with my Granny in the midst of her simple day-to-day life, I learned basic biblical principles. She had a fifth-grade education, but she understood God's Word. She had wisdom and understanding, and she believed by faith. She and my mother had a personal relationship with Jesus Christ. They taught me that we may not understand every detail in God's Word, but that by believing, having faith, and trusting that it's all truth, God will provide and supply all our needs with His understanding and His discernment. That gives me peace that surpasses all human understanding. Philippians 4:7 tells us, "And the peace of God, which transcends all understanding, will guard your hearts and your minds in Christ Jesus." I was taught that we must understand the plan of salvation, because our eternal future depends upon it. There are some things that are revealed to us as we mature and as God chooses to give us the understanding at the time of need. They always said to ask God to guide me and ask for wisdom, and He will always supply my every need. They were exactly right. No wonder the Enemy wanted to cut me off from God and keep me in the desert. He didn't want the next generation to know these valuable teachings. My life's goal is for my children, my grandchildren, and all of the future generations to inherit my love for and desire to know Jesus.

As I grew older and became busy and distracted, I wandered away from God; my spiritual walk weakened. The Enemy knew exactly how to lure me away, and I strayed from all those teachings. The further I wandered into my desert, the more my cravings for materialism and my need for comfort food increased. He knew how to use my old wounds against me; my guard was down, and I was weak. As with Adam and Eve in the garden, the temptation was offered, the lies were told, and the trap was set. They fell and so did I. The hurts from my childhood had been suppressed deep in my heart, causing the process of heart disease to begin. The hurts were not addressed; they were too painful to talk about, they made everyone uncomfortable. Let's just go on with life and forget the past or bury it—that was the strategy. Denial began and old wounds turned into unforgiveness and anger due to my feelings of shame and believing that I was robbed of a normal childhood. At times I felt as if I had been abandoned by God; that was a lie straight from Satan. My childhood pains and anger were becoming adult pains and adult anger, and they hurt even worse. My childhood pains and hurts weren't resolved before I became an adult, so they became displaced. I would release my emotions of anger, sometimes raging on innocent people that I love. My painful emotions became insecurity, dissatisfaction, a dependency on comfort food, and materialism. As a result of my emotional battles, there were consequences to my bad choices, such as unhappiness, obesity, and debt. All these unresolved feelings attacked my self-worth. I was convinced, by the world's perspective, that I needed to get all the nice stuff that all the "normal," happy families possessed, to make me happy and a better person. Nice homes, new cars, expensive clothes, and fad diets could fix me. I soon realized that these were "quick fixes" and only temporary solutions. I was convinced that I could make myself happy and successful. By the world's standards, I was convincingly happy and successful. People could see what was on the outside, that I could achieve and take my rightful place in this world, that I could look good and have lots of "stuff." Only God could see and know the emptiness in the deep cavities of my heart. I had believed all of the Enemy's lies about happiness, what my goals should be for my life and how to get everything that I wanted and so rightly deserved, because God didn't give them to me as a child. I had to get really busy! I allowed Satan to convince me that I was entitled to everything the world has to offer. I began making wrong choices that have resulted in devastating consequences. I had to make up for all the wrong done to me ... me ... me ...! I would make sure that my children would have all the things that I never had and that they would never go without. I wanted to make sure they would be very happy. In the midst of wandering in that desert, it never dawned on me that God had already given me the best life could offer: the simple but valuable spiritual lessons that had been taught to me as a small child. One of which was that I could find some joy and stability in the midst of chaos if I stayed close to God and called upon Him. I overlooked my true blessings because I was blinded by the Enemy's lies. I chose to believe that I had to control and make it right. Oh! God tried to warn me, and he provided direction and ways to turn back, but I ignored His warnings and wandered deeper into my personal desert. My mom tried to warn me about being so busy and wanting too much. I did not heed the warnings, and the day came when, I guess, God decided that He was tired of my grumbling, complaining, and dissatisfaction. So like any good parent, He let me learn from my mistakes and failures. He didn't rush in and fix my life so I wouldn't be uncomfortable. He never deserted me, and He walked with me closely. The evidence of that is that I am able to write all these words contained in this text. God has truly provided everything for me.

My grandmother and my mother have both gone to be with the Lord in heaven, and I am left to fill their shoes to pass on what I have inherited from them: the love, joy, peace, and knowledge of Christ. These are the eternal attributes that will sustain my children and the future generations from Satan's deception. I believe that if intentionally and purposely nurtured, your spiritual foundation will become stronger with each generation.

I married a good man, Thomas M. Pleasants, known to most as Tommy and as "Sealbeam" by his really close graduating friends. He was my high school sweetheart, and we have been through a lot together, some good and some bad. We married very young, and we both recognize that it was due to us wanting to escape from dysfunctional homes. Talking about God's provision, I believe that He placed Tommy in my life, and me in his. I couldn't have found a better soul mate.

Tommy's upbringing was worse than mine. Now, wasn't that a good combination? Kind of like the blind leading the blind. My God is merciful and faithful; He only lets us go to the edge without falling off. He was in control and teaching us along the way. He was always there for us, and He is still with us today, even closer.

Not long after we married, I went back to school and obtained a degree in physical therapy. God opened that door wide, with a job opportunity as a rehab technician, allowing me to be exposed to physical therapy. He provided the way and the finances for me to go back to school; there again, God's provision was very obvious.

7

We bought our first house—small, but nice—and we bought a new car. It too was nice, and I was satisfied for a while. Then "the new wore off," and I had to have a bigger house, a nicer car, and more clothes. My contentment did not last. I used all my stuff for a quick fix, just like an addict. I would gain weight and then lose weight. I needed more clothes or a new hairstyle. Oh, I needed to be more tanned. If my thighs were smaller, I thought, then I would be so happy. I thought a "butt-tuck" might help, but I couldn't afford that, so I determined to buy another exercise machine and work harder to fix my body. The list just goes on and on. I was stuck in another desert. I just kept looking for satisfaction but kept growing more dissatisfied. And let's not forget Tommy; he had his own battles going on with the Enemy. We were about to have a head-on collision. We were both blindly wandering aimlessly, going deeper into our own deserts. God allowed it to teach us about how to be satisfied in Jesus Christ.

The sad thing is that I introduced myself as a Christian. How embarrassing that must have been for God; how I tarnished His image by living a life of overspending, which created a huge amount of debt, seeking pleasure in social drinking and living an undisciplined lifestyle. I knew how to play the game, but God is not a fool, and He will not tolerate disobedience for very long without intervention.

Because of my habitual disobedience, I continued in a cycle of making bad choices. I made choices without asking God's opinion by prayer or by seeking guidance in His Word. I was a little girl looking for satisfaction in the world; I was still empty but filled with guilt. While in this cycle of discontentment, I was completely distracted from any of my spiritual training. If I had focused my energy into strengthening my relationship with Jesus Christ, I would have found satisfaction in His provisions and would not have overlooked the blessings already given to me. I would have stayed out of my deserts by seeking God's will for my life and not have wandered into so many due to Donna's control and plans.

I was preoccupied with working to make more money to meet my many financial obligations and to buy more stuff. The basic simple lessons that kept me safe and grounded in troubled times were completely ignored. In my exhausting efforts in pursuit of the world's expectations and even in the midst of service to God, I continued my fruitless trip into the desert. Proverbs 5:22–23 reads, "The evil deeds of a wicked man ensnare him; the cords of his sin hold him fast. He will die for lack of discipline, led astray by his own great folly." The word "folly" is used to describe our own selfish pursuits of the world. This verse shook my world, and it cut me to the core. It held me accountable! Did I forget to mention that I was a very active, faithful church member? I knew how to practice religion rather than pursue a relationship with Jesus. My church work was even a distraction. I just busied myself to death.

I found myself in a hopeless state, and I was exhausted from no rest and too much worry. I asked what had happened to all my plans and pursuits. I cried out to God, just as my mom had done when our world was falling apart and was out of control. Fear and helplessness can force you to seek help, and I sought God. I prayed and God brought to my memory all the spiritual lessons that were provided for me as a child. The weekends at my Granny Marston's house and the lessons that my mother taught me all came flooding back into my heart. The more I prayed to God, the more I felt filled with an overwhelming sense of peace. God spoke to my heart by the Holy Spirit and assured me that He had everything under control. I was instructed to trust Him and to study His Word for guidance; to start practicing obedience in all areas of my life and living by God's standards and not the world's. He put a desire in my heart to study the "Jesus stories" and restore my relationship with His Son. I found myself going back to the place in my life where I was able to find security and contentment. That place was Granny Marston's house, where and when I felt the presence of Christ. I went back to the times of hearing about the Jesus stories from my mother and my grandmother. I began to read the old, old, stories again, and they were even more meaningful. They were new again. I had a burning desire for Jesus, and to share all His teachings with my children. I wanted to simplify my life and get back to godly basics. I asked God to show me how to start. I had an overwhelming desire to search my heart, to go into those secret places that only God knew about. I was convicted to repent of any unconfessed sin and turn from it. I knew that by doing this, God would start the process of restoration within me, from the inside out. I had faith that He alone would restore what I had allowed Satan to steal from me due to my sin. God placed urgency and a strong need to study His Word and the character of Christ so that I could teach my children and the future generations, just as my mother and grandmother had done for me. To share the knowledge of Christ so that their spiritual walk would be stronger and their wisdom would increase, by doing these things God was making provisions for them. To give them an eternal inheritance that will meet all their needs, a provision that will last forever, even after death. He is always one step or one generation ahead of us.

God has promised that He will never leave or forsake me. My God is a jealous God, and He will not tolerate bad behavior and sin from any of His children. He wants us to be totally dependent upon Him. His Word should be used as our compass to keep us from wandering and becoming trapped in an isolated and barren desert. The Bible is the only standard to be used to evaluate our self-worth and measure our success; not the world's standards because it totally contradicts it.

So this brings me to where I am today. Do I still start to wander? Do I still require accountability? The answer is absolutely yes, because I am human and imperfect. Also, because I am still suffering the consequences of sin, my own and Adam and Eve's, the good news is that I don't wander as far or as often, and I return much, much faster. I am still maturing and growing in Christ. I'm still a "restoration project," and I will not be complete until I die and go to be with God. I just want to share some of the basic spiritual principles that have helped me to resist the temptations and traps set by the Enemy. I'm hoping that sharing parts of my past hurts and present struggles might help you not to wander into a deep, dry desert of no return and end up with a hopeless, destitute lifestyle of habitual sin. I'm hoping and praying that you will seek God, study His Word, and pursue a personal relationship with Jesus. Let's start this journey together, and let's start with using the basic biblical principles that I learned as a small child. They are as easy as A, B, C: Ask ... Believe ... in Christ.

Love in Christ alone, Donna Ashley Pleasants

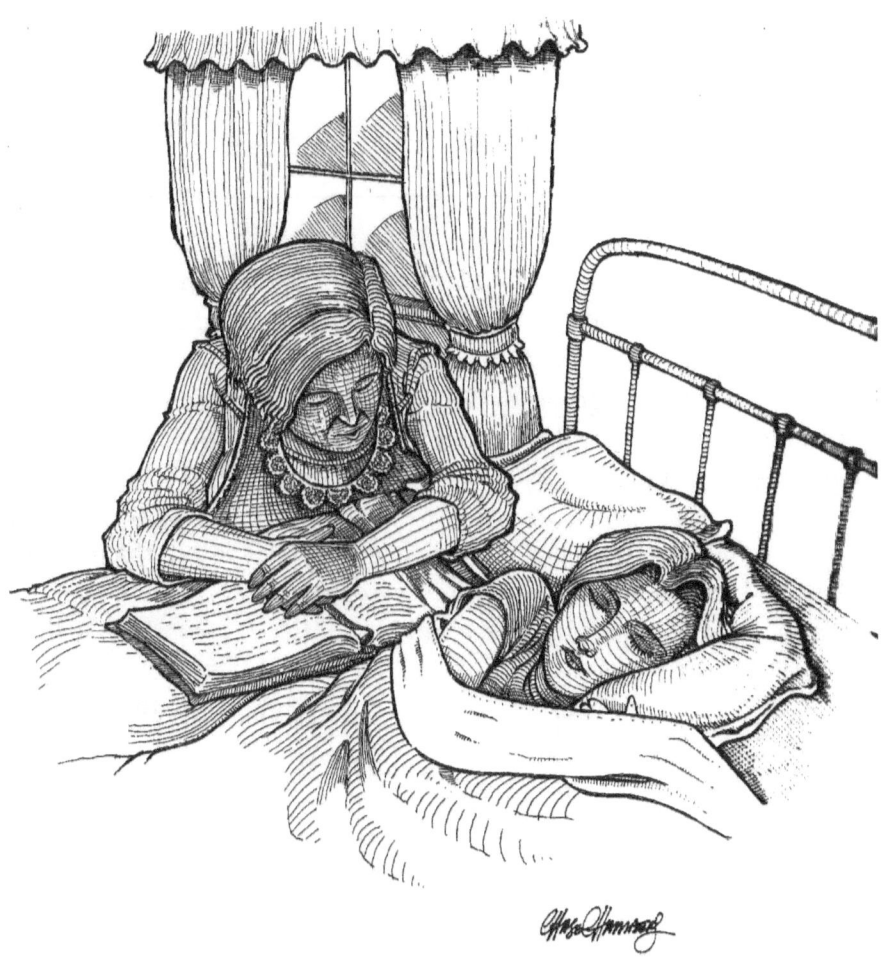

I could hear my Granny Marston call my name while kneeling in prayer.

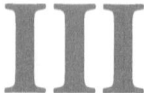

III

MISSION STATEMENT

My mission statement is a reminder that I should become all that God has created me to be and that my life time mission should be to seek Jesus Christ with all my heart, soul and mind. I should attempt to live by His example and share the gospel of Christ to a lost and confused world. It is a reminder that this forty day journey is only the beginning and it will not be finished until I die.

"I'm a restoration project not yet completed until I stand in the presence of God my creator. My life and my body are under restoration in honor of my God, to be used for His service and His glory."

Donna Pleasants

IV

Suggestions for Success and Support

---

1. The New International Bible is to be used for referencing the Scriptures. I have used this version because it is much easier to understand. Please take the time to look up all the scriptures and meditate on them. It will help you to become familiar with your bible and by writing out your answers it will help you to remember them. As you write them view the exercise as if writing them on your heart! For the next 40 days this will play a large part in renewing your mind and starting the restoration process. Be intentional and serious about seeking Jesus to know more about God and His Truth!

2. Pray without ceasing: memorize Romans 12:1–2.

3. Purchase a notebook.

a. Document your journey.

b. Write down prayer requests and answered prayers.

4. Place your forty-day schedule on the refrigerator.

a. Write down your scheduled time to spend with God and pray!

b. Schedule your days to walk.

I recommend brisk walks for thirty to forty-five minutes daily. Incorporate prayer walks with friends or your accountability partner (see below). Listen to Christian music, meditate on His Word, and reflect on Christ's crucifixion, the resurrection, the fruits of the spirit, the parables, the Beatitudes, the Ten Commandments, and the miracles of Jesus. Guard your heart against gossip and idle words. Make your walk about the Creator; look at the creation in awe. Fill your time of walking with praises and positive reflections of your day and life. Choose *joy*.

Praise God and recount all of your blessings. Pray for your enemies and for the lost during your walks. Make your time of exercise and walking be a sacrifice to God, and give it eternal value. Journal your walks.

5. Plan ahead and prepare a menu; intentionally choose healthy foods to prepare for each meal. Plan your meals for a week, and make a shopping list. Purchase only healthy snacks—*no junk food*!

6. Become more active and eat less; cut your amounts in half.

7. Weigh in on the first day that you begin your journey. That will be the start of this study. Don't weigh again until you finish your forty-day commitment. Don't focus on weight loss, numbers and the external, but focus on making internal changes by the renewing of your mind. Eternal changes comes from the inside out and will last forever.

8. Commit yourself for forty days to start your process of restoration by seeking God and studying His Word. Ask God to expose anything in the secret places of your heart that will keep leading you back into your personal desert. Start making the lifestyle changes that will impact your spiritual and physical health, by the process of renewing your mind.

Let's get out of our personal deserts!

This is not a quick fix or a "miracle diet" solution. Again, it is about choosing to renew our minds for making lifestyle changes that will affect all areas of our lives, including our spiritual growth, our finances, our appearance, and our health. There are rewards for practicing and living with discipline, self-control, and obedience as our standards; these are requirements for balance established by God.

Change needs to take place from the inside out, starting with our thoughts; everything starts in the mind. That is why it is so important to renew our minds with the instruction and knowledge of God's Word. Change begins with our thoughts, which are then processed with our hearts. The condition of our hearts will determine how we respond to practicing discipline and obedience to God's Word and authority. If our hearts are pure and filled with a love for God, our appetites and cravings for fulfillment will gradually change. We will begin to desire less of what the world has to offer for a quick fix. "Therefore, prepare your minds for action, be self-controlled; set your hope fully on the grace to be given you when Jesus Christ is revealed.

As obedient children, do not conform to the evil desires you had when you lived in ignorance" (1 Peter 1:13–14).

If we ask, God will give us the understanding and knowledge of His Word to equip us to achieve our goals, to live by His standards, and to bring permanent change into our lives. We must pray, asking with pure hearts and pure motives that will glorify God. Making our motives all about pleasing God will give us the strength and ability to succeed.

Commit to making the necessary changes by applying the spiritual and physical A, B, C, principles. Make the choice of renewing your mind daily, and start the process of change in your life for the next forty days. The Lord kept the Israelites in the desert for forty years (read Numbers 32:13). Jesus was sent out into the desert for forty days (read Mark 1:12–13). The number forty is significant in the Scriptures, so let us start with the number

God used. Let's totally commit to start the process of renewing our minds for the next forty days.

Choose an accountability partner who is serious about making lifestyle changes. Choose someone who will commit to focus on prayer and to seek God's will, someone who will use this study as a guide to starting the process of renewal and restoration. Remember, the process will be a lifetime commitment.

Pray for each other to overcome your personal deserts. It could be a spiritual problem, a financial burden, overeating, or some other addiction. Whatever your personal desert might be, commit to finding your way out for the next forty days. Hold each other accountable to achieve the goal. Don't miss a single day of commitment, regardless of any temptation that will come against you. You must choose to intentionally put on your armor for protection against any attack, whether it is of the flesh or from Satan.

We must pray by faith and believe that God will answer, pray without ceasing to begin our forty-day journey strong. We must also continue to pray to finish our forty-day journey with a deeper relationship with Jesus Christ, which will equip us to finish our lifelong journey even stronger!

"Finally, be strong in the Lord and in His mighty power" (Ephesians 6:10).

V

Start with a Strong Foundation

Before we begin our process of restoration, let's examine our spiritual foundation—that foundation being our relationship with Jesus Christ. In any structure, a weak foundation will collapse under stress or strain. The same applies to our lives. If we know Jesus as our personal Savior and truly know His character, our foundation will be strong. That strong personal relationship will be our cornerstone, and we will be equipped to withstand all the trials of life. It is not enough to just know the name; we must know Jesus the person.

Are you absolutely sure that you know Jesus Christ as your personal Lord and Savior? If you died at this very moment, would you be in the presence of your Holy God? If your answer is, "I hope so," or "I think so," then you don't have the assurance and security of genuine salvation. If you question your salvation, don't hesitate to talk with someone. Please don't wait! Talk with someone immediately; don't put it off for another second. This is the most important decision of your life; where you spend eternity depends upon it. If you have any doubts, ask someone to pray with you. If you have never prayed the prayer of salvation to receive Christ as your Lord and Savior, do it now. If you have the security and peace that comes from having a deep personal relationship with Jesus, you'll have a strong foundation for the process of restoration to begin.

"Consequently, you are no longer foreigners and aliens, but fellow citizens with God's people and members of God's household, built on the foundation of the apostles and prophets, with Christ Jesus as the chief cornerstone. In Him the whole building is joined together and rises to become a holy temple in the Lord. And in Him you too are being built together to become a dwelling in which God lives by his spirit" (Ephesians 2:19–22).

Steps to Receive Christ

1. Confess any sin in your life (past and present).

2. Repent and ask God for forgiveness.

3. Turn from your sin—*stop it!*

4. Ask Jesus to dwell in your heart, and earnestly seek a relationship with Him.

5. Profess that Jesus is the Son of God, that he was crucified on the cross, and was buried, and that on the third day he arose from the dead. Believe that the Holy Spirit resides within your heart.

6. Pray and ask for wisdom and understanding of God's Word, and seek a deep relationship with Jesus Christ. "For God so loved the world that He gave his one and only Son that whoever believes in Him shall not perish but have eternal life" (John 3:16).

Congratulations! If you prayed this prayer and accepted Jesus as your Lord and Savior, you are a new creature in Christ. You now have the freedom to live the life for which you were created, freed from sin, to serve God the Father and to experience the eternal joy of Christ. You now are a child of God, come to the Father with childlike faith. Seek God with all your heart; come to know Him as your Creator and your Father. Come to know Jesus as the Son and your Savior. Come to know the Holy Spirit as your counselor and as God's sweet voice. Continue to pray and listen for him to speak. Get involved in a community of believers, attend a strong Bible-teaching church, and study and meditate on the Word of God. Prayerfully seek the truth for your life, and be obedient to God's plan.

Read and meditate on the meaning of these Scriptures.

Ask for wisdom and understanding. "Therefore, if anyone is in Christ, he is a new creation; the old has gone, the new has come!" 2 Corinthians 5:17

John 14:15–17: "If you love me, you will obey what I command. And I will ask the Father and he will give you another Counselor to be with you forever—the Spirit of truth. The world cannot accept him, because it neither sees him nor knows him. But you know him, for he lives with you and will be in you."

VI

THE SIGNIFICANCE OF THE NUMBER FORTY

God's Word is the one book of authority we should use as our standard for living. All the words were written by ordinary men called by God to do extraordinary things through obedience. They were inspired and empowered by God, and they found His will for their lives. The Bible says that all the words are "God breathed and are useful for teaching, rebuking, correcting and training." I try to pay special attention to any words, phrases, or numbers that are repeated in the Scriptures. I believe that if God repeats something, it must be extremely important and for our benefit. How many times have we had to repeat warnings or instructions to our children before they got it?

One number I have noticed repeatedly is forty. I have observed that the number forty usually relates to a length of service, fasting, praying, teaching, rebuking, specific measurements, or judgment. This is why I have chosen that particular number of days for our total commitment to start our process of restoration. To start strong and to be successful, we must totally commit to seek God for forty days. To begin this process of change, we must read and study the Scriptures in this guide and learn to apply all the basic A, B, C, principles for spiritual and physical training. Let's look closely at the number forty and some of the ways that God used it through His written Word.

In your Bible find and read the passages below, include verses before and after to give you an understanding of each verse. Then fill in each blank.

1. Genesis 7:4

"Seven days from now I will send rain on the earth for _____ days and _____ nights, and I will wipe from the face of the earth every living creature I have made."

2. Exodus 16:35

"The Israelites ate manna _____ years, until they came to a land that was settled, they ate manna until they reached the border of Canaan."

3. Exodus 24:18

"Then Moses entered the cloud as he went on up the mountain. And he stayed on the mountain _____ days and _____ nights."

4. Exodus 34:28

"Moses was there with the Lord _____ days and _____ nights without eating break or drinking water. And he wrote on the tablets the words of the covenant—the Ten Commandments."

5. Numbers 13:25

"At the end of _____ days they returned from exploring the land." (Numbers 13:25).

6. Numbers 14:33–34

"Your children will be shepherds here for _____ years, suffering for your unfaithfulness, until the last of your bodies lies in the desert. For _____ years—one year for each of the _____ days you explored the land—you will suffer for your sins and know what it is like to have me against you."

7. Deuteronomy 25: 2–3

"If the guilty man deserves to be beaten, the judge shall make him lie down and have him flogged in his presence with the numbers of lashes his crime deserves, but he must not give him more than _____lashes. If he is flogged more than that, your brother will be degraded in your eyes."

8. Judges 3:11

"So the land had peace for _____ years, until Othniel, son of Kenaz died." (Judges 3:11)

9. Judges 5:31

"So may all your enemies perish, O Lord! But may they who love you be like the sun when it rises in it's strength." Then the land had peace _____ years.

10. Judges 8:28

"Thus Midian was subdued before the Israelites and did not raise its head again.During Gideon's lifetime, the land enjoyed peace _____ years."

11. Judges 13:1

"Again the Israelites did evil in the eyes of the Lord, so the Lord delivered them into the hands of the Philistines for _____ years."

12. 1 Samuel 4:18

"When he mentioned the ark of God, Eli fell backward off his chair by the side of the gate. His neck was broken and he died, for he was an old man and heavy. He had led Israel _____ years."

13. 1 Samuel 17:14-16

"David was the youngest. The three oldest followed Saul, but David went back and forth from Saul to tend his father's sheep at Bethlehem. For _____days the Philistine came forward every morning and evening and took his stand."

14. 2 Samuel 5:4

"David was thirty years old when he became king, and he reined _____years."

15. 1 Kings 11:42

"Solomon reigned in Jerusalem over all Israel _____years."

16. 1 Kings 2:10–12

"Then David rested with his fathers and was buried in the City of David. He had reigned _____ years over Israel-seven years in Hebron and thirty years in Jerusalem."

17. 1 Kings 6:14–17

"So Solomon built the temple and completed it. He lined its interior walls with cedar boards, paneling them from the floor of the temple to the ceiling, and covered the floor of the temple with planks of pine. He partitioned off twenty cubits at the rear of the temple with cedar boards from floor to ceiling to form within the temple an inner sanctuary, the Most Holy Place. The main hall in front of this room was _____cubits long."

18. 1 Kings 19:8

"So he got up and ate and drank. Strengthened by that food, he traveled _____ days and _____ nights until he reached Horeb, the mountain of God."

19. Ezekiel 41:2

"The entrance was ten cubits wide, and the projecting walls on each side of it were five cubits wide. He also measured the outer sanctuary; it was _____ cubits long and twenty cubits wide."

20. Ezekiel 4:6

"After you have finished this, lie down again, this time on your right side, and bear the sin of the house of Judah. I have assigned _____ days, a day for each year."

21. 2 Kings 12:1

"In the seventh year of Jehu, Joash became king, and he reigned in Jerusalem _____ years."

22. Ezekiel 29:11–12

"No foot of man or animal will pass through it; no one will live there for _____ years. I will make the land of Egypt desolate among devastated lands, and her cities will lie desolate _____ years among ruined cities. And I will disperse the Egyptians among the nations and scatter them through the countries."

23. Jonah 3:4

"On the first day, Jonah started into the city. He proclaimed:"_____ more days and Nineveh will be overturned."

24. Matthew 4:1-2

"Then Jesus was led by the Spirit into the desert to be tempted by the devil. After fasting _____days and _____nights, he was hungry."

25. Acts 13:21

"Then the people asked for a king, and he gave them Saul son of Kish, of the tribe of Benjamin, who ruled for _____ years."

26. Acts 1:3

"After his suffering he showed himself to these men and gave many convincing proofs that he was alive. He appeared to them over a period of _____ days and spoke about the Kingdom of God."

27. Acts 7:30

"After _____ years had passed, an angel appeared to Moses in the flames of a burning bush in the desert near Mount Sinai." .

The number forty, as you have just seen, is used a lot in the Old Testament and less in the New Testament. I'm not sure why, but if I had to guess, I would say that maybe after the birth of Jesus, people were more accepting, more obedient, and more faithful to God.

Let's move forward and go deeper into the Word of God. Let's get excited about the changes that will come from the inside out by renewing our minds. Remember ask and believe He will answer, thank Him ahead of time, by faith!

VII

ARE WE ANY DIFFERENT THAN THE ISRAELITES?

The book of Exodus explains how Moses was called and directed by God to lead the Israelites out of the bondage of slavery. They were permitted to leave Egypt after God directed Moses to declare a series of plagues upon Egypt and Pharaoh.

The Israelites are identified as God's chosen people, but they were also a rebellious people. They were so rebellious and disobedient that God allowed them to wander in the desert for forty years. God did not forsake them, and it wasn't His plan for them, but it was the consequence of their sin. Can't we identify with them? How much time do we spend wandering in our own personal deserts, which are created by our own rebellion and disobedience? How often do we wander further and further away from God, grumbling and complaining, never being satisfied? God's protection and provision were available to them, but they continued to rebel, and their hearts turned away from Him. Do we still do this today? It should have taken the Israelites 11 days to make their journey to the promised land but because of their disobedience it took them much, much longer.

It took forty years, and God used that time to teach and train His children in His ways."And we know that in all things God works for the good of those who love him, who have been called according to his purpose" (Romans 8:28).

God miraculously provided and led them out of the desert into the Promised Land of Canaan. But before they were allowed into the Promised Land, the land of milk and honey, Moses had to remind them of all the miraculous things that God had done for them. Do *we* have to be reminded of what God has done for each of us? Do we also quickly forget?

The Israelites also had to be reminded that they were chosen by God for His covenant, and so had to obey the laws of God. *Covenant* means a binding agreement between two or more people. God promised to deliver the Israelites out of Egypt into the land of plenty, and His people were to love Him and keep His laws. In the Old Testament, a blood sacrifice such as an unblemished lamb or goat was offered up to God in atonement for human sins. They were to live out the covenant with God. I have to ask myself, *What is keeping me from entering into my own promised land of milk and honey? What desert am I stuck in because I am not in a covenant relationship with God? Is my disobedience going to cause me to wander for 40 years or longer?*

> Give thanks to the Lord, call on His name; make known among the nations what He has done. Sing to Him, sing praise to Him, tell of all His wonderful acts. Glory to His holy name; let the hearts of those who seek the Lord rejoice. Look to the Lord and His strength; seek His face always. Remember, the wonders He has done, His miracles, and the judgments He pronounced. O descendants of Israel His servant, O sons of Jacob, His chosen ones. He is the Lord our God; His judgments are in all the earth. He remembers His covenant forever, the word commanded for a thousand generations. (1 Chronicles 16:8–15)

God provided for and protected the Israelites because Moses remained faithful and interceded for them.

Read Deuteronomy 9:7–29 from your Bible. Look closely at verses 16 and 19. What was Moses' response when he saw God's chosen people sinning against God? They had made a golden calf to worship, and they clearly had turned from the way of the Lord.Read verse 18; what did Moses do in behalf of his sinful people?

Read Deuteronomy 9:19 again, and then fill in the blanks.

I _____the _____and _____of the Lord, for he was _____enough with _____to _____ you. But again the Lord _____ to me.

Thank God, Moses interceded and was obedient with fasting and petition of prayer. He was overwhelmed with burden for the Israelites, and he pleaded with God to save them from themselves. Have *we* ever been so burdened or afraid for another person because of their sins? To the point that we fall prostrate before the Lord for even one night, much less for forty days and nights?

Moses gave us an example of accountability and intercessory prayer to which has been given for each of us to follow. Who might be praying for you? More importantly, whom are you interceding for?

The Ten Commandments were given to Moses for his people to pattern and govern their lives according to God's standard. God's commandments are not just a set of rules. They were given as a design to give direction and with the purpose of discerning right from wrong. Disobedience to the Word of God brings failure and punishment. Obedience to the Word of God brings prosperity and blessings. Obedience produces peace.

In the New Testament, God makes a new covenant with His people. No longer is there a need for a blood sacrifice of animals to atone for sin. He gave us His son, Jesus, as the ultimate sacrifice and the atonement for all sin, past and present. We can't earn or buy salvation; all we have to do is accept and believe the truth, which is Jesus Christ! "For this reason, Christ is the mediator of a new covenant, that those who are called may receive the promised eternal inheritance, now that he has died as a ransom to set them free from the sins committed under the first covenant." Hebrews 9:15

If we totally trust and obey God, we are promised deliverance and salvation, which comes by believing in Jesus Christ, which will produce the fruits of the spirit, and we will find eternal rest.

God's Word will never change, and He will keep His sovereign promises. Yes, we can be forgiven, but there will be consequences of our disobedience. This is why God gives us warnings throughout His Word. The ones that He repeats throughout the Scriptures should make us stop and examine our lives and surrender to His authority.

We do not have to fear and worry about anything that we might encounter on life's journey, because our relationship with Jesus Christ is enough to overcome any consequence, even death. He conquered every adversity, including His crucifixion and death. Jesus paid the debt for our sins; He came to seek and save the lost. Today we are in a new covenant relationship with God because of the blood that Jesus shed upon the cross in payment for all of our sins. "For the Son of Man came to seek and save what was lost." Luke 19:10.

Read below and put your name in the blank space provided.

For the Son of Man came to seek and to save _____ who was lost.

Amen! Thank your Father for your provision of salvation so that you may have eternal life if you simply Ask and Believe in Christ!

VIII

THE CALL

By faith I have accepted Jesus Christ as my personal Lord and Savior. I *believe* that Jesus is very much alive and at work in my life. I am not perfect, and I don't claim to be even close to that. "For all have sinned and fall short of the glory of God, and are justified freely by His grace through the redemption that came by Christ Jesus" (Romans 3:23–24). I fall short of the glory of God every day, but I do recognize that I am forgiven and can change.

God's faithfulness and mercy bring me out of the deserts that I wander into when I am disobedient and out of His will. I pray that this simple study will assist you to start seeking wisdom and an understanding of God's Word. I encourage you to seek His Word and discover the mysteries hidden there for each of His children to find when they so desperately need the counsel of a loving father.

What a precious gift to be able to experience the Father's love through the gift of His living Word, which was prepared thousands of years ago for such a time as this! "And who knows but that you have come to royal position for such a time as this?" (Esther 4:14).

I pray that you will not be afraid to knock on the door to a place of hope, forgiveness, and rest. *Ask* with confidence that it be opened to receive Christ into your heart. *Believe* that Christ will open the door and welcome you into His Father's house. Jesus says: "Ask and it will be given to you; seek and you will find; knock and the door will be opened to you. For everyone who asks receives; he who seeks finds; and to him who knocks, the door will be opened" Matthew 7:7–8. And in John 14:2–4, Jesus tells us: "In my Father's house are many rooms; if it were not so, I would have told you. I am going there to prepare a place for you. And if I go and prepare a place for you, I will come back and take you with me that you also may be where I am. You know the way to the place where I am going."

This is where we will begin our journey to the Father's house, but, before we begin restoration, we must identify the issues or sins that keep us out of God's will. His Word can help us identify some of the deep-rooted problems within our hearts. I speak not of the physical heart but of the spiritual heart. I believe, however, that they are closely intertwined. It takes balance to be spiritually and physically healthy. Balance is a direct result of order and discipline. Please don't think that I don't struggle with balance. This is just one area of my life in need of change, as revealed to my heart by the Word of God. I feel deeply convicted to share what I have experienced and learned about God with others that might be in need of encouragement and accountability.

My hope is that God will use these writings to bring glory to Himself and help you look inward and identify sin, such as unforgiveness and anger. I pray that you can find healing to your past hurts and pains, and that restoration may occur by drawing closer to and developing a personal relationship with the Son. God's Word tells us that we can come to God the Father only through our relationship with Jesus the Son. Jesus said, "I am the way and the truth and the life. No one comes to the Father except through me" John 14:6.

The word *journey* is often used to refer to the human life. According to Webster's, it means traveling to one place to another, not remaining in the same place, to keep moving. To grow and mature spiritually, you have to be actively involved in a relationship with Jesus Christ and progressing forward with maturity in the knowledge and understanding of God's Word. In physical training you have to be actively involved in an exercise program, progressing forward as your muscles strengthen and your endurance levels change. Choosing to remain in your present condition and not moving or progressing forward will not strengthen you spiritually or physically. You will become comfortable in your present condition, whether spiritual or physical, until trauma or sickness occurs, and then you are forced to make changes in your life. Our journeys' paths and progress are determined by our choices of direction, discipline, and obedience.

Because of my disobedience and lack of discipline, I have made my journey (life) harder and far more complicated than my Father God intended. There are many areas of my life that have been affected by the emotional issues of my childhood, but the two most significant areas are emotional eating and emotional spending. I know God is going to address all the issues that have allowed Satan to rob me of my spiritual blessings. In my spiritual weakness I allowed sin to slowly creep into my life, and I lost my direction. I have been led to share my life experiences with other women and to explain how our spiritual condition could predetermine our physical health. I am a licensed physical therapy assistant, and I am licensed to teach structured exercise and endurance training programs. I have been practicing physical therapy for over thirty-five years. Because of my background and knowledge of exercise and human anatomy, I was approached by several ladies in our church to lead an exercise class. We successfully continued the class for over ten years. Many passed through the class, but the core, committed group remained faithful. I believe this is due to our prayer time, our discipline, and our accountability to one another; we developed strong relationships. The thing I've heard most over the years is the need for change: the change for a better life, for better health,to lose weight and for the need of being satisfied. They were just "sick and tired of being sick and tired."

The purpose and plan for my life was set in motion when I committed to help these ladies start an exercise class. I began to teach them about their bodies and explain how God has uniquely created each of them for a greater purpose. We discussed how we have to be spiritually and physically prepared to fulfill that purpose. Little did I know of the profound effect their needs would have on me. I began looking inward and seeking God to understand why so many of us had the same needs and complaints about ourselves, why so many of us were so dissatisfied.

I realized there was a lot about myself that I needed to change before I could help anyone else. At that time I was about fifty pounds overweight and very unhappy with my appearance. It's taken years for me to come to the realization that how I look should not determine my degree of happiness. I've learned by prayer and reading God's Word that true satisfaction and joy come from the inside. True joy and satisfaction come only by a deep relationship with Jesus. My motivation and focus had been totally wrong and self-centered. That is why all of my yo-yo diets and material possessions never gave me lasting satisfaction. I always looked for a quick fix. God revealed to me that I should focus on my spiritual condition more than on my physical looks, by developing spiritual disciplines; the transformation would come from the inside out. (Romans 12:1–2). I believe that God sees our obedience and discipline as a sacrifice and will honor that as an offering of giving up self. My motivation changed, and I worked harder to stay on the right path. My motivation turned from being self-centered to the understanding of the Scriptures.

"Therefore, I urge you, brothers, in view of God's mercy, to offer your bodies as living sacrifices, holy and pleasing to God—this is your spiritual act of worship. Do not conform any longer to the pattern of this world, but be transformed by the renewing of your mind" Romans 12:1–2. My mind is in the process of being renewed by feeding on God's Word and digesting it. It is not a one-time deal; it is a daily, moment-by-moment process. The renewal of my mind and thoughts has changed my cravings from physical comfort food to spiritual food for eternal nourishment. It's what I have been "hungering" for all my life; I developed a hunger for Jesus Christ.

During this process I realized that I had buried some of my childhood pains under layers of unforgiveness. This kept my focus on me.

I do believe that we should be concerned about our bodies and appearance, because we are representatives of God. We should have a desire to protect our health and try to look our best but not be consumed or controlled by an obsession. My obsession with my weight and appearance kept me in bondage. My biggest concern was what the world could see with its physical eyes, and I did not consider how my Father God was hurt by what He saw deep in the secret places of my heart with His spiritual eyes.

"Train a child in the way he should go, and when he is old he will not turn from it" Proverbs 22:6. I always believed this verse was intended to be used for training my children, but God revealed that he has applied this passage to my whole life. God had been training me, His child, throughout my life's journey. He allowed me to wander in the desert to teach me. He applied the loving discipline that was necessary to mature my faith. The Father's love prevailed, and it will for His disobedient and rebellious children. Our Father has given us instructions and commands to follow to make our journey good and joyful.

What are your thoughts or beliefs about the Ten Commandments? Define *commandment*:

_____

_____

_____

_____

_____

The word *commandment* means a command, an order, a mandate or law. Why has God given us the Ten Commandments? Do you believe they are intended to be a set of rules to restrict us from the freedom of enjoying our lives? Can you see how they actually set us free from living under the bondage of fear, and how they set boundaries that provide freedom? Like any good parent, God set boundaries for His children—not to harm us, but to keep us safe. When Adam and Eve introduced sin to the world by their disobedience, God had to have a plan that would provide limitations for his children to follow for stability and structure. God had set the example for perfect parenting. When children are disobedient, discipline is required for correction, just as God has done with the past generations and will continue with the future generations, for as long as the world exists.

Looking at the world and local news broadcasts, it appears there are many people that do not know the commandments. Do you believe they still apply to our lives today, or do you believe they were written for the people who lived thousands of years ago? Explain your thoughts.

_____

_____

_____

_____

_____

_____

_____

If the Ten Commandments came from God, why are they being removed from the sight of his people? Explain your thoughts.

_____

_____

_____

_____

_____

_____

As believers in the Word of God, what is our responsibility to restore the value of the Ten Commandments in society today?

_____

_____

_____

_____

_____

_____

_____

_____

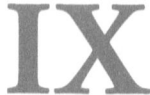

IX

THE TEN COMMANDMENTS

Read Exodus 20:1–17.

And God spoke all these words: "I am the Lord your God who brought you out of Egypt , out of the land of slavery."Exodus 20:1-2

1. "You shall have no other gods before Me." Exodus 20:3

2. "You shall not make for yourself an idol in the form of anything in heaven above or on the earth beneath or in the waters below. You shall not bow down to them or worship them; for I, the Lord your God, am a jealous God, punishing the children for the sin of the fathers to the third and fourth generation of those who hate me, but showing love to a thousand generations of those who love and keep my commandments." Exodus 20:4-6

3. "You shall not misuse the name of the Lord your God, for the Lord will not hold anyone guiltless who misuses His name."Exodus 20:7

4. "Remember the Sabbath day by keeping it holy. Six days you shall labor and do all your work, but the seventh day is a Sabbath to the Lord your God. On it you shall not do any work, neither you, nor your son or daughter, nor your manservant or maidservant, nor your animals, nor the alien within your gates. For in six days the Lord made the heavens and the earth, the sea, and all that is in them, but he rested on the

seventh day. Therefore, the Lord blessed the Sabbath day and made it Holy."Exodus 20:8-11

5. "Honor your father and your mother, so that you may live long in the land the Lord your God is giving you: Exodus 20:12

6. "You shall not murder.' Exodus 20:13

7. "You shall not commit adultery." Exodus 20:14

8. "You shall not steal." Exodus 20:15

9. "You shall not give false testimony against your neighbor." Exodus 20:16

10. "You shall not covet your neighbor's house. You shall not covet your neighbor's wife, or his manservant or maidservant, his ox or donkey, or anything that belongs to your neighbor."Exodus 20:17

Do you believe that there are serious consequences for those that choose to break or ignore God's commandments?

Read Ecclesiastes 12:13 in your Bible. Why would we be warned to fear God if there were no consequences of not keeping His commands? God is a God of love, but Scripture supports and clearly indicates that He has expectations for His children and that there are consequences to disobedience; He will not tolerate anyone's sin.

Read Ecclesiastes 12:14 in your Bible. It clearly states that God will bring every deed, good or bad, into judgment.

Read Isaiah 13:9–13 in your Bible. I know in these passages that the prophet Isaiah is referring to Babylon and warns Babylon to turn from its wickedness. Read these passages and apply them to yourself; make them personal and apply them to the condition of your home.

Do you have peace in your heart, or do you feel anxious after reading these Scriptures? Pray for God to reveal the areas of your life that need correction; ask for forgiveness for your disobedience.

Are the Ten Commandments being lost with each generation today, or are they being made known to each generation today? Look at the condition of our nation for evidence to support your answer.

_____

_____

_____

_____

We are either obedient or disobedient children. Can the Ten Commandments be compromised? Explain.

_____

_____

_____

_____

_____

Do you understand that breaking a commandment is direct disobedience to God? If so, why?

_____

_____

_____

_____

_____

_____

Read the Ten Commandments again, and remember that God's Word cannot be compromised. What are you doing right now that is causing you to be directly disobedient to God's authority?

_____

_____

_____

_____

According to the Word of God, what will be the consequence of continuing in habitual sin? Write your answer in the space below. You will be forgiven, but disobedience *will* result with consequences. It does not matter who you are or how many possessions you have; God will judge your disobedience!

_____

_____

_____

_____

God is our authority of the most high, and to ignore His commandments is rebellion against Him. Read Romans 13:1–5. Pay close attention to verses 1 and 2; now rewrite them in your own words, and make them personal.

_____

_____

_____

_____

_____

_____

Read James 3:1-12 Is it possible to commit murder with our words?In the spaces provided express your thoughts.

_____

_____

_____

Can you honestly say that you don't steal? Examine all areas of your life, including time and service. What might we be stealing from God?

_____

_____

_____

_____

_____

_____

Are there any of the Ten Commandments that you might struggle with keeping? Dr. Henry Blackaby teaches in the Bible study, "Experiencing God," that partial obedience is disobedience. Do you understand this concept?" If so, write out your understanding.

_____

_____

_____

Do you believe that the condition of your heart could be the source of your struggle with keeping God's commandments? Read Isaiah 6:8–10, it's greater to have "heart knowledge" than to have "head knowledge."

In the space below, write out your understanding of verses 9 and 10. Explain how this will strengthen you so that you can be more obedient to God's commands.

_____

_____

_____

_____

_____

The scriptures often speaks of having "wisdom", read James 3:13-18. It describes two sources of "wisdom", in the spaces provided identify the two sources and their characteristics. Which do you identify with?

_____

_____

_____

_____

_____

_____

_____

_____

Do you understand that what you "harbor" in your heart effects your obedience to God's word?

_____

_____

What does the word *rebellion* mean? It means to resist or oppose authority. I can remember as a teenager being rebellious of my parents' authority. That was direct disobedience to God's authority. I broke the command to honor my father and mother. The command doesn't say to honor and obey if they are perfect parents. God gives the command without any occasion for argument.

My disobedience caused my parents and myself much pain. My rebellion led not only to disobedience but to consequences that followed. It is the same with God, our Father, when we rebel against his Word or authority; it grieves His heart and it forces Him to apply discipline for correction. He has to hold us accountable for our actions so that we can be refined, and to bring change into our lives. He always forgives, but He doesn't always remove the consequences; he exemplifies perfect parenting. Study and pray over the Ten Commandments, and ask God to reveal any rebellion or disobedience in your heart. Pray with your accountability partner, and choose to walk in obedience to God's Word. Our degree of obedience and submission to God's Word reflects how much we love God. Jesus said: "Whoever has my commands and obeys them, he is the one who loves me. He who loves me will be loved by my Father, and I too will love them and show myself to him" (John 14:21). And in 1 John 5:3 we read, "This is love for God: to obey his commands. And his commands are not burdensome, for everyone born of God overcomes the world. This is the victory that has overcome the world, even our faith. Who is it that overcomes the world? Only he who believes that Jesus is the son of God."

Continue to study and clothe yourself with God's Word, and know that I am interceding for each person that reads this material to receive the understanding with their heart. "Make the heart of his people calloused; make their ears dull and close their eyes. Otherwise they might see with their eyes, hear with their ears, understand with their hearts, and turn and be healed." Isaiah 6:10

X

Spiritual A, B, Cs ... Ask, Believe in Christ, Restored by Truth

A.... Ask

Ask and it will be given to you, seek and you will find, knock and the door will be opened to you.

—Matthew 7:7

When you ask, you do not receive because you ask with wrong motives that you may spend what you get on your pleasures.

—James 4:3

Ask in prayer for God to reveal what is suppressed in that empty cavity of your heart. Old hurts and childhood pains can cause your heart to be diseased. For years I have suffered from the dreaded disease of discontentment and dissatisfaction. I've been in the medical field for over thirty-five years, and I relate to medical analogies. A cardiac surgeon can open up a chest cavity and examine the human heart with his or her eyes, but only God can examine someone's spiritual heart. He knows what is hidden in that secret place, and you can't hide it from Him!

Read Hebrews 3:7–15, focusing on verse 12. This verse gives a clear warning about what causes a hardened heart. Read Hebrews 3:12 again, and fill in the blanks below:

"See to it, brothers, that _____ of you has a _____ _____,
heart that _____ away from the _____ God. Hebrews." 3:12

What was the consequence of their rebellion that caused them to have hardened hearts? Read Hebrews 3:11, and fill in the blank.

So I declared an oath in my anger, "They shall _____ enter my rest." (Hebrews 3:11).

Who made this declaration? _____

What does it mean not to be able to enter into God's rest?

_____

_____

Read Hebrews 3:13–14. We are being instructed to encourage one another daily, so that we are not to be deceived and fall into sin and disbelief, causing our hearts to be hardened. We are to share Christ with one another and to believe with the utmost confidence that the Word of God is absolute truth and given for each of us to follow and obey.

What is meant by the word truth, according to John 3:21, John 8:31–32, John 14:6–7, and Hebrews 10:26–27?

Write out the meaning of each verse in your own words, and share them with your accountability partner.

_____
_____
_____
_____
_____
_____
_____
_____

How will you know the truth unless you study the truth? To know the truth is to be free in Christ Jesus.

Read Hebrews 3:7–8 and Hebrews 3:15 again. They are exactly the same; both verses are warnings. For them to be given twice in the same chapter, they must be very important to God. He doesn't want us to miss this instruction. He is trying to warn us and prevent us from developing hardened hearts.

Read Hebrews 3:16–19. Are we rebelling against the Word of God today, just as people did thousands of years ago? Do His Word and warnings apply to us today?

Disobedience to God's authority that is clearly stated and explained in his written Word will surely be dealt with as individuals and in groups today. His Word applied to the people thousands of years ago, and it applies to people today. His Word never changes.

Obedience comes from accepting the Word of God as truth by faith and believing in God's sovereignty and unfailing love for all people.

Read Hebrews 3:18. Whom did God keep from entering His rest?

_____

_____

Why were they unable to enter His rest?

_____

_____

Being able to enter into God's rest is very important, because that rest gives us the assurance that God is in control and will keep all of His promises. His rest is eternal. God's rest is the hope that is given by knowing Jesus Christ and is the peace that will keep us grounded. Obedience and submission to God's authority will allow us to experience His rest even in the midst of the most difficult storm. I choose to believe this by faith, because it is a promise from the Almighty God.

B...Believe

Then Jesus cried out, "When a man believes in me, he does not believe in me only, but in the one who sent me. When he looks at me, he sees the one who sent me. I have come into the world as a light, so that no one who believes in me should stay in darkness." John 12:44–46 Have you ever asked, who is God? To find the answer to this question this scripture clearly directs us to look at and study Jesus. By faith we are to believe everything the scriptures say about him and by doing this you come to know God!

Believe that the Word of God is 100 percent truth, and that the Word of God is "God breathed." In your Bible, read John 1:14, which states that "the Word became flesh." To whom does this refer?

_____

_____

_____

Read John 1:1 and fill in the blanks below:

"In the beginning was the _____, and the Word _____ _____ God, and the _____ was _____."

The word *believe* means to accept as truth, to have trust or confidence in a statement or promise of another person. To believe the Word of God means that you truly trust in God the person. Before you can trust someone or what they say, you first have to know them and have a relationship with them. The only way to trust and know a person is by spending time with them, then you can believe what that person says and except it as absolute truth. The only way to know God is to spend time with Him in prayer and by reading His word. Faith is developed and strengthened as you apply the scriptures to your daily life and discover the power that comes from the resource directly from God!

Believe that the Scriptures are alive and are directly from God, given to humankind for wisdom and guidance throughout our earthly lives. Don't just read the Word for head knowledge; meditate on the Scriptures and know them in your heart, and make them personal. Believe every word!

Psalm 19:14: May the words of my mouth and the meditation of my heart be pleasing in your sight, O Lord, my rock and my redeemer.

Proverbs 4:20–22: "My son, pay attention to what I say; listen closely to my words. Do not let them out of your sight; keep them within your heart, for they are life to those who find them and health to a man's whole body ."

Job 22:22–23: "Accept instruction from his mouth and lay up his words in your heart. If you return to the Almighty, you will be restored."

Romans 10:10: "For it is with your heart that you believe and are justified, and it is with your mouth that you confess and are saved."

Psalm 119:105: "Your word is a lamp to my feet and a light for my path."

Let the words of God guide you out of your personal desert. Pray with your accountability partner to stay on God's path and to remain in His will, especially for the next forty days.

Make the appropriate changes in your life that will reflect the standard of God's Word. Approach the Scriptures with a childlike faith. "I tell you the truth, unless you change and become like little children, you will never enter the kingdom of heaven. Therefore, whoever humbles himself like this child is the greatest in the kingdom of heaven" (Matthew 18:3–4).

John 20:29: Then Jesus told him, "Because you have seen me, you have believed, blessed are those who have not seen and yet have believed."

John 20:31: "But these are written that you may believe that Jesus Christ, the Son of God, and that by believing you may have life in his name."

John 11:40: Then Jesus said, "Did I not tell you that if you believe, you would see the glory of God?"

Acts 16:31"Believe in the Lord Jesus Christ, and you will be saved."
James 1:1-2 Consider it pure joy, my brothers, whenever you face trials
of many kinds, because you know that the testing of your faith develops
perseverance. Perseverance must finish its work so that you may be mature
and complete, not lacking anything. If any of you lacks wisdom, he should
ask God, who gives generously to all without finding fault, and it will be
given to him. But when he asks, he must BELIEVE and not doubt, because
he who doubts is like a wave of the sea, blown and tossed by the wind.

Have faith and believe and live out the Word of God. Faith means having
an unquestionable belief in God.

Find each passage in your Bible, and fill in the blanks below:

2 Corinthians 5:7

"We live by _____, not by sight."

Romans 3:22

"This righteousness from God comes through _____ in Jesus
Christ to all who believe."

Romans 5:1

"Therefore, since we have been justified through _____, we have peace
with God through our Lord Jesus Christ, through whom we have gained
access by _____ into this grace in which we now stand. And we
rejoice in the hope of the glory of God."

Romans 10:17

"Consequently, _____ comes from hearing the message, and the
message is heard through the word of Christ."

1 Corinthians 16:13

"Be on your guard; stand firm in the _____; be men of courage; be strong."

Galatians 2:20

"I have been crucified with Christ and I no longer live, but Christ lives in me. The life I live in the body, I live by _____ in the Son of God, who loved me and gave himself for me."

Hebrews 11:1

"Now _____ is being sure of what we hope for and certain of what we do not see."

Hebrews 11:6

"And without _____ it is impossible to please God, because anyone who comes to him must believe that he exists and he rewards those who earnestly seek him."

Believe and have faith that all that is written in the Holy Bible is a clear reflection of God's heart and that it is the living truth. Meditate on and study His words; develop heart knowledge to be filled and satisfied.

How often should we meditate on His Word? Read Psalm 119:97–99. Verse 97 says that we should "meditate on it all day long." Verses 98 and 99 state that by meditating on God's Word, we will become wiser and have more insight, with a better understanding, which will give a great desire to be more obedient, which will in turn increase our faith and help our unbelief.

In your Bible read Matthew 17:14–20. Read the first part of verse 17 again, and fill in the blank below. Jesus said, "O _____ and perverse generation." In verse 19, the disciples asked Jesus why they could not heal the boy of the demon. In verse 20 He explained why: "Because you have so little faith. I tell you the truth, if you have faith as small as a mustard seed, you can say to this mountain. Move from here to there and it will move. Nothing will be impossible for you."

Now turn to Matthew 21, and read verses 18–22. Read verses 21 and 22 again, and fill in the blanks below.

Jesus replied, "I tell you the truth, if _____ have _____ and _____ _____ doubt, not only _____ you _____ what was done to the fig tree, but also _____ _____say to this mountain, "Go, throw yourself into the sea, and it be done."

"If _____ _____, _____ _____receive whatever you _____for in _____."

Jesus wants us to have faith and believe that He is the Son of God. He wants to use us to accomplish great things, because He is now with the Father. His motive is to bring glory to God and to show mankind that He is still alive and at work. Only by our obedience can this be accomplished. Read John 14:11–14 below.

> "Believe me when I say that I am the Father and the Father is in me; or at least believe on the evidence of the miracles themselves. I tell you the truth, anyone who has faith in me will do what I have been doing. He will do even greater things than these, because I am going to the Father. And I will do whatever you ask in my name, so that the Son may bring glory to the Father. You may ask me for anything in my name, and I will do it."

Believe that Jesus can and will do it! You can't have faith without belief!

Read the passages below, and meditate on what they say about the heart.

Psalm 51:10 "Create in me a pure heart, O God, and renew a steadfast spirit within me."

Psalm 119:32: "I run in the path of your commands, for you have set my heart free."

1 Chronicles 28:9 "And you, my son Solomon, acknowledge the God of your Father, and serve him with whole- hearted devotion and with a willing mind, for the Lord searches every heart and understands every motive behind the thoughts. If you seek Him, He will be found by you; but if you forsake Him, He will reject you forever."

1 Samuel 16:7: "But the Lord said to Samuel, Do not consider his appearance or his height, for I have rejected him. The Lord does not look at the things man looks at. Man looks at the outward appearance, but the Lord looks at the heart."

Luke 16:15: "You are the ones who justify yourselves in the eyes of men, but God knows your hearts. What is highly valued among men is detestable in God's sight."

Colossians 3:1: "Since, then you have been raised with Christ, set your hearts on things above, where Christ is seated at the right hand of God."

John 14:1: "Do not let your hearts be troubled. Trust in God; trust also in me."

Romans 10:10: "For it is with your heart that you believe and are justified, and it is with your mouth that you confess and are saved."

Matthew 6:21: "For where your treasure is, there your heart will be also."

Proverbs 4:23: "Above all else, guard your heart, for it is the wellspring of life."

Deuteronomy 11:18: "Fix these words of mine in your hearts and minds."

Matthew 5:8: "Blessed are the pure in heart, for they will see God."

Ezekiel 36:26–27: "I will give you a new heart and put a new spirit in you; I will remove from you your heart of stone and give you a heart of flesh.

And I will put my spirit in you and move you to follow my decrees and be careful to keep my laws."

Ask God to expose the true condition of your heart. Are you suffering from a diseased heart? Does that deep-rooted something (sin) keep you captive or in bondage? Is there something that you are clinging to or a "stronghold" that keeps you going deeper into that same old desert?

Are you in a cycle of indulging in yo-yo diets, overspending, or obsession with your appearance? Are you in a state of dissatisfaction? Are you constantly making the wrong choices by following your heart's desire for temporary pleasure?

Maybe you are not even aware of what is the real problem. Is it so painful that you have suppressed it to the point that it is not identifiable? Could it be anger, unforgiveness, lying, greed, deception, or addictions, including food, shopping, or work?

Have you hardened your heart? Have disobedience and rebellion become your lifestyle, which has become very comfortable and natural? Have you been deceived to believe that all your sin is justified and that there is no other way to live or to conduct your business? Has your heart become so hardened that the Word of God does not penetrate it, and you can barely hear His voice anymore? Have you worn yourself out because you are not allowed to enter into God's rest because of your disobedience? If you can't find peace and are unable to let your soul and mind rest, you will weaken spiritually; eventually, you will not even have physical rest. The Enemy will deceive you and use your sin against you. Whatever you choose to bury and hold on to will become a stronghold. Sin will make you a slave. Read in your Bible Romans 6:16–23. Then read verse 16 again; what is the consequence of being a slave to sin?

_____

What is the reward for obedience? _____

Read Romans 6:20 again, and fill in the blanks below.

"When you were _____ to _____, you were _____ from the control of _____."

In your Bible, read Galatians 6:7–8, and then read Romans 6:21 again.

Galatians 6:7 says, "Do not be deceived: God cannot be mocked. A man reaps what he sows."

According to Romans 6:21, what does a person reap from sin? _____

According to Galatians 6:8, what does a person reap from obedience or living to please God? _____

According to Romans 6:22, what is the benefit and what will be the result of being set free from sin? _____ and _____

"For the wages of sin is death, but the gift of God is eternal life in Christ Jesus our Lord" (Romans 6:23). This verse makes clear our choices: death or eternal life. Which of the two do you choose?

Ask God in prayer for guidance, instruction, and for an understanding of his Word. *Believe* that you will receive, and God will open the door for you to enter into His rest. Matthew 7:7–8 instructs us: "Ask and it will be given to you; seek and you will find; knock and the door will be opened to you. For everyone who asks receives; he who seeks finds; and to him who knocks the door will be opened."

C...Christ

Christ was given to us to study, to be our role model. He is to be the pattern in developing our character. Christ can restore and heal. This is why He was sent to live among us. "But he was pierced for our transgressions, he was crushed for our iniquities, the punishment that brought us peace was upon him, by his wounds we are healed" (Isaiah 53:5).

We are going to study the character of Christ and come to know Him in a deeper personal relationship. So much is written about Jesus in the teachable experiences of his life. His response to his life's experiences exposes his undiseased heart! It reveals the depth of his connection to His heavenly Father's heart. His deep unconditional love is also revealed in how He responded to so many personalities and problems. The source of His peace is shown to us by his response to His life's challenges and relationships. He lived as a man being confronted with difficult people with many trials. He counseled many hurting people experiencing different types of pain, including death. He could heal the sick and even raise the dead.

He shows us how to love unconditionally and how to exhibit compassion even to the least desirable. He is a resource of unlimited hope, the Great Physician, and a counselor; and He brings light into a darkened world tarnished by sin. Thank you, God, for sending your Son, our Savior.

Let's learn more about Jesus' undiseased heart and how by knowing and believing in Him, our diseased (sinful) hearts can be healed.

In Matthew, chapter 5, Jesus called His disciples to come and sit with Him on the side of a mountain. This was an invitation for them to spend time with Him. I believe that Jesus purposely chose a mountainside, to further emphasize the powerful teachings that they were about to receive from God Himself. Have you ever stood on the side of a mountain and been overwhelmed by the breathtaking view? What a majestic picture of creation, and what a visual example of God's creative power. Maybe Jesus felt closer to His Father on that mountainside. Can you imagine sitting on that beautiful majestic mountainside listening to the Son of the living God, knowing that the man that was teaching you was actually the Son of the very God that created that mountain!

This invitation is known as Jesus' Sermon on the Mount, wherein Jesus gave the disciples the Beatitudes. The Beatitudes were the pronouncements given by Jesus for God's blessings to be received. They were given to the disciples on that day to reveal and to expose God's pure heart, and also for our daily application to heal our hearts.

By accepting that invitation, they learned more about the Son of God and became more personally involved with Him. Jesus is still giving that invitation to each of us today. He wants us to come to Him, to sit with Him, to pray and to study God's Word, to listen and to learn more about Him. We are to develop a pure, intimate relationship with the Son of God, so that we can imitate His character. He wants to teach us about His Father's love and how we are to love the Father enough to live a life of obedience, which will bring glory to God. Jesus has shown us, by His obedience, all the way to the cross, how to deeply love the Father and how to seek His will, even unto death.

Let's turn to Matthew 5:1–11. These are the intentional teachings that our Savior wanted to leave with His disciples, but He also was thinking about us, the future generations that would have to believe by faith and not by sight. Jesus knew His time was short, and He used every situation and every opportunity to teach about God. He did not care about what people thought; He came to seek and to save the lost. Shouldn't this be the same attitude in each of us? He sat with prostitutes, He ate with tax collectors, and He spent time with the lepers. His motives were pure, and everything He did was out of obedience to His heavenly Father. Jesus did not approve sin; he was always the accountability and gave an answer of how to stop sin. Who do we spend time with, friends, co-workers and family? Due to our love for them and because God's expectation of obedience are we able to hold them accountable to sin? Does fear of "offending" them keep us from leading them to Jesus and eternal life?

Each of the Beatitudes reveals the heart of God the Father, and also of Jesus the Son. Read each one below. Can you identify with each one?

The Beatitudes: Matthew 5:1–11

Now when He saw the crowds, He went up on a mountainside and sat down. His disciples came to Him and He began to teach them saying: (Matthew 5:1-2)

"Blessed are the poor in spirit, for theirs is the kingdom of heaven."(Matthew 5:3)

"Blessed are those who mourn for they will be comforted."(Matthew 5:4)

"Blessed are the meek, for they will inherit the earth."(Matthew 5:5)

"Blessed are those who hunger and thirst for righteousness, for they will be filled."(Matthew 5:6)

"Blessed are the merciful, for they will be shown mercy."(Matthew 5:7)

"Blessed are the pure in heart, for they will see God."(Matthew 5:8)

"Blessed are the peacemakers, for they will be called sons of God."(Matthew 5:9)

"Blessed are those who are persecuted because of righteousness, for theirs is the kingdom of heaven."(Matthew 5:10)

"Blessed are you when people insult you, persecute you and falsely say all kinds of evil against you because of me."(Matthew 5:11)

Each of the Beatitudes has a deep, personal truth about God's heart and character, and they reveal His expectations of His children. They are given to us so that we can have new hearts. We should embrace the Beatitudes and clothe ourselves with them until we are transformed into His likeness. We must be imitators of Christ so that we can be equipped to live a life of discernment and obedience that will enable God to work in us and through us.

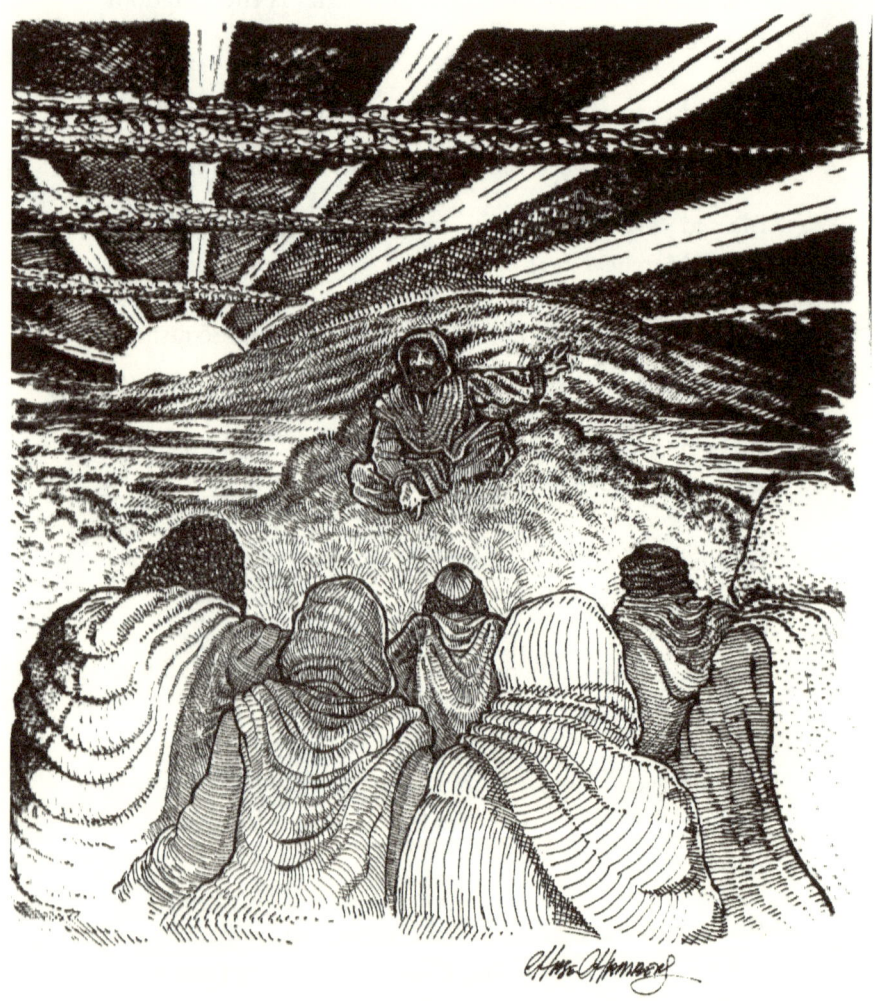

Jesus teaching his disciples The Beatitudes.

Read the verses below with your accountability partner, and pray for God to reveal the characteristics of Christ. Write them in the spaces provided.

Galatians 5:22–26 _____

_____

_____

1 John 3:16 _____

_____

_____

John 3:13–15 _____

_____

_____

Isaiah 53:5–7 _____

_____

_____

Luke 2:8–12 _____

_____

_____

John 14:6 _____

_____

Pray for your accountability partner and yourself to be disciplined and committed for the next forty days. Pray for the renewal of your mind and that you will be transformed into the image of Christ. Through this process, God can heal and restore you.

Read the Scriptures listed below, and meditate on each; feed upon them and digest them. Internalize their meaning and seek to find what valuable lessons are revealed. Pray that you will develop an understanding of the words of God in each passage. Ask for the truths of each verse to be revealed to you and that you will develop heart knowledge, not just head knowledge. Pray for the understanding of each verse and how it is to be applied to your daily life. Continue to pray for the next forty days that you will be transformed by the renewing of your mind. Pray also that you will begin to live by the control of the Holy Spirit and by this principle you will develop the discipline and the character of Christ. Renew your mind and satisfy your hunger by "feasting" on the "fruit of the Spirit".

Turn to Galatians 5 and read verses 16 through 25, and fill in the blanks provided:

So I say, live by the Spirit, and you will not gratify the desires of the sinful nature. For the sinful nature desires what is _____ to the _____ and the Spirit what is _____ to the _____ _____. They are in _____ with each other, so that you do _____ do what you _____. But if you are led by the _____, you are not under law. The acts of sinful nature are obvious;_____ immorality, _____ and _____; _____ and _____; hatred, _____, _____, fits of _____, _____ ambition, dissensions, factions and envy; drunkenness, _____ and the like. I warn you, as I did before, that those who live like this _____ _____ _____ the _____ of _____. But the fruit of the _____ is _____, _____, _____, _____, _____, _____, _____, _____ and self-_____. Against such things there is no law. Those who belong to _____ _____ have _____ the _____ nature and with its _____ and _____. Since we _____ by the _____, let us keep in step with the _____.

List the fruits of the spirit that describe Christ:

1.

2.

3.

4.

5.

6.

7.

8.

9.

Which do you struggle with? Pray and ask God to show you why. Explain.

_____

_____

_____

_____

_____

_____

_____

_____

_____

_____

Read verse 24 again, and explain what this verse means to you.

_____

_____

_____

_____

_____

_____

_____

Read verse 25 again, and explain what this verse means to you.

_____

_____

_____

_____

_____

_____

Read the verses below and seek the lessons of each one. Evaluate each situation and look for the fruits of the spirit. What was Jesus' interaction with and response to each need? Everything that Jesus said and did was intentional and for a specific purpose. That purpose was to reveal and teach something about God by His responses. In the spaces provided, write your understanding of each passage and what you learned from each one. Answer with your heart, not just from your head. Note: These accounts are also recorded in the book of Luke.

Matthew 8:1–4: Jesus heals a man with leprosy.

_____

_____

_____

_____

_____

_____

Matthew 8:5–13: Jesus heals a centurion's servant.

_____

_____

_____

_____

_____

Matthew 8:14–17: Jesus heals Peter's mother-in-law.

_____

_____

_____

_____

_____

_____

_____

_____

_____

Matthew 8:23–27: Jesus calms the storm.

_____

_____

_____

_____

_____

Matthew 8:28–34: Jesus sends demons into a herd of pigs.

_____

_____

_____

_____

_____

Matthew 9:1–8: A paralytic is healed.

_____

_____

_____

_____

_____

_____

Matthew 9:18–33: A ruler's daughter is brought back to life; a woman is healed of a bleeding disease; Jesus heals the blind and a mute.

_____

_____

_____

_____

_____

_____

Matthew 14:13–21: Jesus feeds five thousand.

_____

_____

_____

_____

_____

_____

Matthew 14:22–33: Jesus walks on water.

_____

_____

_____

_____

_____

These miraculous stories of Jesus and how He healed many people and helped them overcome impossible human situations give us a clear picture of God's compassion. The stories reveal what is required of us to experience Him and also reveal His power. I don't think we understand what a gift his power is to us. "A wise man has great power, and a man of knowledge increases strength." Proverbs 24:5

That strength is obtained by having heart knowledge and understanding of the Word of God, and through completely trusting by faith that the Bible contains all that we need to overcome any problem. We are to believe that having a personal relationship with the Son of God gives us access to an unlimited source of power to overcome any of Satan's schemes, and the power to have victory over any circumstance. That power comes directly from God. Read the Scriptures below, and underline the word *power*. Also underline the source of the power:

1. Matthew 22:29: Jesus said, "You are in error because you do not know the scriptures or the power of God."

2. Acts 1:8: Jesus said, "But you will receive power when the Holy Spirit comes on you ..."

3. Acts 10:38: John preached of how God anointed Jesus of Nazareth with the Holy Spirit and power ...

4. Colossians 1:10–12: And we pray this in order that you may live a life worthy of the Lord and may please him in every way; bearing fruit in every good work, growing in the knowledge of God, being strengthened with all power according to his glorious might so that you may have great endurance and patience, and joyfully giving thanks to the Father ...

5. Hebrews 1:3: The son is the radiance of God's glory and the exact representation of his being, sustaining all things by his powerful word …

6. 2 Corinthians 12:9: Jesus said, My grace is sufficient for you, for my power is made perfect in weakness."

7. Philippians 3:10:" I want to know Christ and the power of his resurrection and the fellowship of sharing in his suffering, becoming like him in his death."

God the Father was the source of power that raised Jesus from the dead. Knowing Jesus the person and having a personal relationship with Him will enable us to endure the sufferings that we will experience in our lives. For us to become like Him in His death, we will have to be totally submissive to God, and totally selfless. As a child of God, that power is given to us by knowing God the Father and His Word, having a personal relationship with his Son, Jesus Christ, and by the leading of the Holy Spirit which empowers us to sustain our peace in the midst of life's storms and to overcome and "defeat" Satan!

Christ, while on earth as a man, was able to relate to various types of people with serious problems and limitations. He was a storyteller who could communicate biblical teachings simply. His style was so simple that a child could understand it. He was very effective thousands of years ago, and by the Scriptures and the Holy Spirit, he remains effective today. I know this to be true, because when I was a small child in need, my blessed mother and grandmother told me the parables and about the miracles of Jesus. As I have mentioned, I called them the Jesus stories. I never forgot these, and I came to know and love Jesus Christ in a very real way. As a small child, I could not verbally explain everything, but I knew Him in my heart. I trusted and believed with a childlike faith. He met my needs then and continues to meet my needs today. When I was a little girl, my mother taught me a precious little song. I accepted that chorus as an invitation for Jesus to come into my heart. We sang it as a prayer: "Into my heart, into my heart, come into my heart, Lord Jesus. Come in today, come in to stay. Come into my heart, Lord Jesus."

I sang that precious song with a genuine devotion and desire for this person, Jesus, to come and actually dwell in my heart. I couldn't explain how it happens, but I knew from all the evidence that I had heard about this man that He was real, and He was able to fill my heart with whatever I needed. That was my real acceptance of Christ, by my childlike faith.

As a child, when things around me seemed to be falling apart, I knew Jesus was with me. For example, I experienced His peace by remembering the story of Him walking on the water in the midst of a terrible storm. The disciples were in a boat, and they were very afraid. Jesus told Peter to get out of the boat and walk to Him. Peter obeyed and started walking toward Jesus. He was able to walk on water as long as He believed and kept his eyes on Jesus. That story was simple enough for me to understand, and it gave me a picture and an understanding of God's Word.

My faith and my knowledge of Christ matured as the years passed, but I will never forget the Jesus stories or that sweet little song. Jesus came into my heart and will remain there forever. The Jesus stories continue to give me peace, hope, and an understanding of how to apply my faith. As long as I continue to keep my eyes fixed upon Him, I will not sink! Amen!

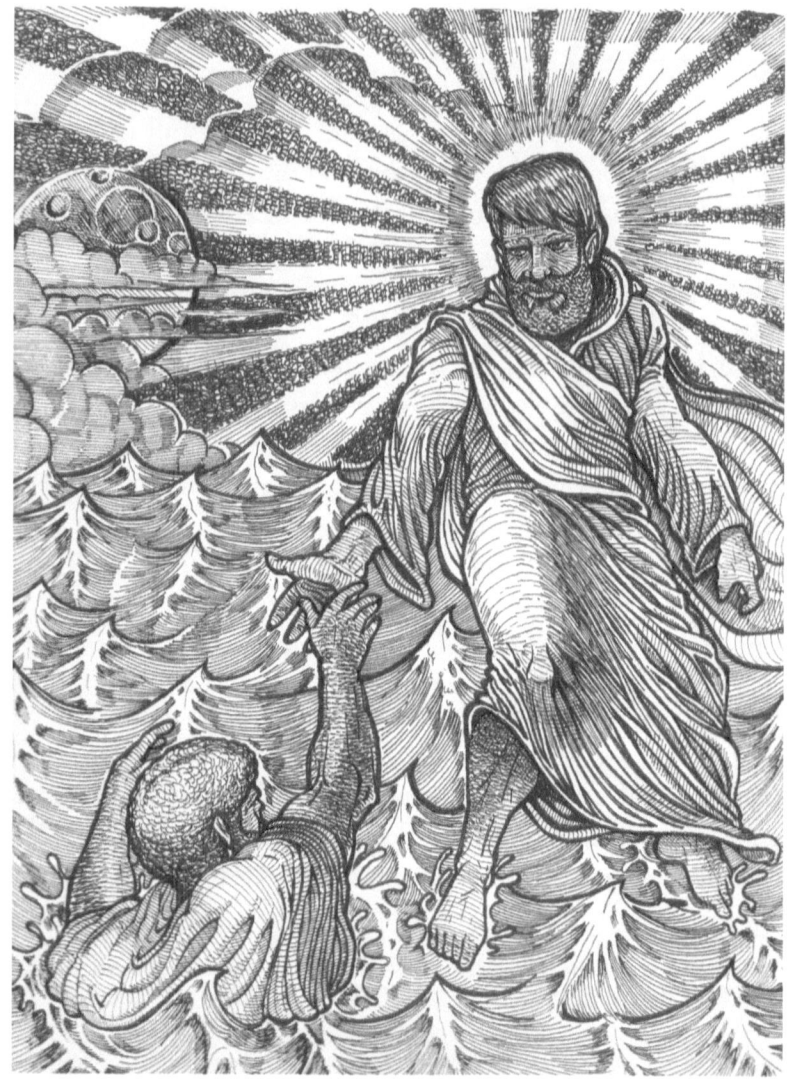

"You of little faith", Jesus said,"why did you doubt?" Matthew 14:31

"I will open my mouth in parables; I will utter hidden things, things from old" (Psalm 78:2). Jesus spoke to many in parables; what a counselor He was and is today. He wants us to think and find a way to apply His practical teachings, to be intentional about revealing His character by how we live.

A parable is a short allegory that teaches a moral. An allegory is a story in which characters and actions are symbols for ideas or ideas to symbolize the actual meaning of something. God used parables to draw us deeper into the Word and He used them in an intentional and unique way to spark our interest to seek the truths for their value and understanding. God is so creative!

How can parables be used in developing our Christlike character so that we can be used by God?

Read each of the parables, and write out the hidden truth and application of each one.

❖

Matthew 13:1–23: The Sower

_____

_____

_____

_____

_____

_____

_____

❖

Matthew 13:24–30: The Wheat and the Weeds

_____

_____

_____

_____

_____

_____

_____

❖

Matthew 13:31–32 The Mustard Seed

_____

_____

_____

_____

_____

_____

❖

Matthew 13:33–35: The Yeast

_____

_____

_____

_____

_____

❖

Matthew 13:36–43: The Weeds in the Fields

_____

_____

_____

_____

_____

❖

Matthew 13:44–46: The Hidden Treasure and the Pearl

_____

_____

_____
_____
_____
_____
_____

❖

Matthew 18:10–14: The Lost Sheep

_____
_____
_____
_____
_____
_____

❖

Matthew 19:16–30: The Rich Young Ruler

_____
_____
_____
_____
_____
_____

❖

Matthew 20:1–16: A Land Owner Hiring Workers

_____
_____
_____
_____

_____

_____

_____

❖

Matthew 21:33–46: The Wretched Tenants

_____

_____

_____

_____

_____

_____

❖

Matthew 22:1–14: The Wedding Banquet

_____

_____

_____

_____

_____

_____

❖

Matthew 25:1–13: The Ten Virgins

_____

_____

_____

_____

_____

_____

❖

Matthew 25:14–30: The Talents

_____

_____

_____

_____

_____

_____

_____

Matthew 21:28–32 The Parable of the Two Sons

_____

_____

_____

_____

_____

_____

_____

Matthew19:13–15 The Little Children and Jesus

_____

_____

_____

_____

_____

_____

_____

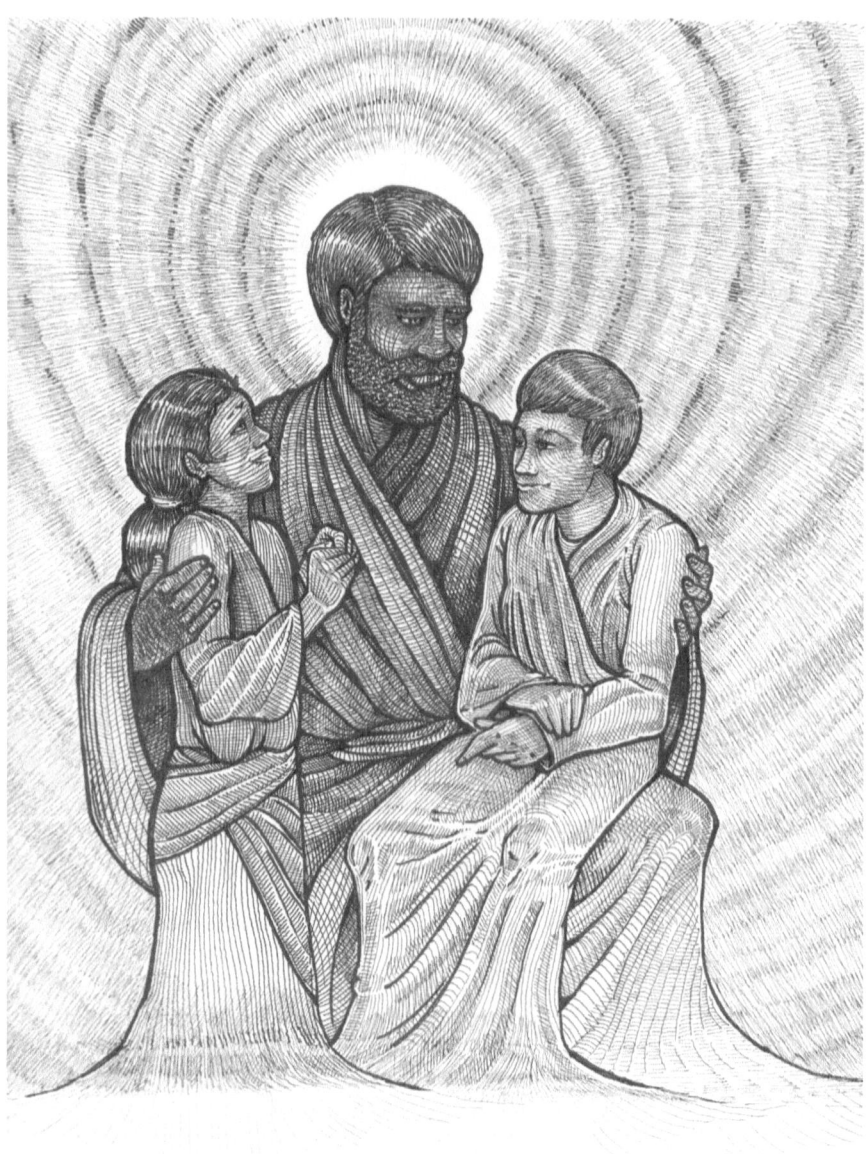

Jesus said, "Let the little children come to me, and do not hinder them, for the kingdom of heaven belongs to such as these." Matthew 19:14

Matthew 18:15–20 A Brother Who Sins against You

_____

_____

_____

_____

_____

_____

_____

Matthew 18:21–35 The Parable of the Unmerciful Servant

_____

_____

_____

_____

_____

_____

_____

Matthew 22:34–40 The Greatest Commandment

_____

_____

_____

_____

_____

_____

_____

Do you understand and see the value of each of these teachings? Explain your answer.

_____

_____

_____

_____

_____

_____

_____

Do you believe that if they are applied to your everyday living and interjected into your relationship with people, internal change will take place? Explain your answer.

_____

_____

_____

_____

If you adapt and apply the teachings from the parables into your daily living, who will people see?

_____

In the space below, explain what you believe about the parables and why.

_____

_____

_____

_____

_____

_____

_____

Why do you think Jesus spoke in parables?

_____

_____

_____

_____

_____

_____

When Jesus spoke He always spoke clearly and with simplicity; it was as if He was talking to and teaching children. He knew that in some situations He had one chance to impact a person or a crowd. He purposely and intentionally had "eternal conversations." Jesus taught with simplicity and a heart for saving souls.

Change is hard for most of us, and it requires stepping out of your comfort zone into unfamiliar territory and having to rely on trust, faith, and accountability. In other words, we need help from our Christian brothers and sisters. They are to help us stay on the right path and not return to the comfort of "going back into the wilderness or our desert."

Read James 5:16, and meditate on the emphasis on God instructing each of us to have accountability. "Therefore confess your sins to each other and pray for each other so that you may be healed." The prayer of a righteous man is powerful and effective."

Accountability is a very important element for our Christian character to be stable. We are to be held accountable by the standard of God's Word, the Holy Spirit, and by fellow Christians. Our fellow Christians are not to judge, but they are to hear our confessions of sin, to warn us about the sin in our lives, and to pray with us. Their prayers are to strengthen and to encourage us to stay within God's will. Our Christian brothers and sisters are to help guide us and keep us out of our personal deserts.

Meditate and study the teachings in this study for the next forty days. Allow God's word to hold yourself and your accountability partner accountable to His standard. Walk with each other, and reflect on how the Holy Spirit has spoken to each of you. Continue to pray for the renewal of your mind, remembering that it's a process.

Pray for your heart to be restored, and by that restoration you will find your way out of your personal desert. The truth will be your compass and guide for eternity.

I pray that you will keep focused and recycle all the teachings in this study until your Christian journey becomes easier as you develop and practice discipline in all areas of your life, which will result in balance. Restoration is a process and it will not be completed until we die and meet our Creator face to face. It is then when we each will be held accountable for our entire life.

Hebrews 4:13: Nothing in all creation is hidden from God's sight. Everything is uncovered and laid bare before the eyes of Him to whom we must give account.

Romans 14:9–12: For this very reason, Christ died and returned to life so that He might be the Lord of both the dead and the living. You, then, why do you judge your brother? Or why do you look down on your brother? For we will all stand before God's judgment seat. It is written, "As surely as I live, says the Lord, every knee will bow before me; every tongue will confess to God." So then, each of us will give an account of himself to God.

So as the Holy Spirit says, "Today if you hear His voice do not harden your heart as you did in the rebellion during the time of testing in the desert" (Hebrews 3:7).

The desert can represent a time in your life where you experience very difficult problems and situations, so difficult that you have felt isolated and alone, with an overwhelming sense of hopelessness. Do you see yourself in a time of testing or in a personal desert?

In your Bible, read Hebrews 3:8. What is the warning? _____

_____

The word *rebellion* means an act or state of armed, open resistance to authority or defiance of any control. To resist God's authority or to rebel against Him is disobedience.

Read Romans 13:1–2: "Everyone must submit to the governing authorities, for there is no authority except that which God has established. The authorities that exist have been established by God. Consequently, he who rebels against the authority is rebelling against what God has instituted, and those who do so will bring judgment on themselves."

According to God's Word in Romans 13, verse 2, what happens if we are disobedient and rebellious against His authority?

_____

_____

_____

_____

_____

_____

_____

Disobedience or rebellion brings discipline or punishment that is given for correction and direction, because of a deep, sincere love from a holy and just God.

How do we keep from drifting away and becoming rebellious? Read Hebrews 2:1–3 in your Bible. Verse 1 tells us that we must pay more careful attention to what we have heard, so that we do not drift away. There are two key words in this passage. The first is "must," which means it is absolutely necessary. The second is "careful," which warns us to be cautious and intentional. It is essential that we pay very close attention to who and what?

Turn to Hebrews, chapter 1, and read verses 1–3, paying close attention to verse 2. It says: "The Son is the radiance of God's glory and the exact representation of His being, sustaining all things by His powerful word." It is essential to pay close attention to the Son, because He is God, and His Word is the power that keeps us in His will of obedience. Therefore, we will not drift away from God's authority.

Jesus Christ is the only source of eternal light and is the everlasting hope coming directly from God's glory. He was sent into a world that has been darkened by sin. Read John 3:16–18: "For God so loved the world that He gave His one and only son, that whoever believes in Him shall not perish but have eternal life. For God did not send His son into the world to condemn the world, but to save the world through Him. Whoever believes in Him is not condemned, but whoever does not believe stands condemned already because he has not believed in the name of God's one and only son" (John 3:16–18).

If a man lives in the light, he will have no shame. But if a man rejects the truth and remains in darkness, he will hide and isolate himself for fear of being exposed. We may hide our lies and corruption from family, friends, and community, but nothing can be hidden from the almighty God!

Read John 3:19–21: "This is the verdict: Light has come into the world, but men loved darkness instead of light because their deeds were evil. Everyone who does evil hates the light, and will not come into the light for fear that his deeds will be exposed. But whoever lives by the truth comes into the light, so that it may be seen plainly that what he has done has been done through God. "

Only by paying close attention to the instructions in God's Word and intentionally choosing to apply them to our daily lives can we keep from straying from our relationship with Jesus. If you know the Son, you will know and experience the Father. God's holy Word is the only thing that will sustain us and keep us from failing.

Read Hebrews 4:6–13: "It still remains that some will enter that rest, and those who formerly had the gospel preached to them did not go in because of their disobedience. Therefore, God again set a certain day, calling it Today, when a long time later He spoke through David, as was said before: "Today, if you hear His voice, do not harden your hearts". For if Joshua had given them rest, God would not have spoken later about another day.

There remains, then, a Sabbath—rest for the people of God; for anyone who enters God's rest also from his own work; just as God did from His. Let us, therefore, make every effort to enter that rest, so that no one will fall by following their example of disobedience. For the word of God is living and active. Sharper than any double-edged sword, it penetrates even to divide soul and spirit, joints and marrow; it judges the thoughts and attitudes of the heart. Nothing in all creation is hidden from God's sight. Everything is uncovered and laid bare before the eyes of Him to whom we must give an account." Let's look at what these verses are saying. What is the significance of Today being capitalized in verse 7? It states "Therefore God set a certain day, calling it Today, when a long time later he spoke through David, as was said before: "Today, if you hear his voice, do not harden your hearts." I believe God is warning us if we have heard the gospel and it is of no value to us and we do not apply it by faith and we continue in our sin, He will not give us rest. We will not experience rest on earth or eternal rest after death. Today is the day of knowing Jesus Christ! Jesus should be the Lord of our life and He alone gives us rest. Jesus is Today!

Again, we are warned not to harden our hearts by disobedience. If the Holy Spirit speaks, we must obey or face the consequences for our sin. Read verse 11 again. It plainly states that if we are disobedient we will fall and may cause others to fall.

Read verse 12. What about the heart is being judged?

_____

_____

_____

_____

_____

Read verse 13 again. Pay close attention to the deep meaning of each word of this verse. It should cause us to tremble to know that nothing is hidden from the almighty and powerful God and that all will be laid bare before His eyes. Each of us will give an account for our disobedience. Knowing that I will literally stand before the most holy God, the creator of humans, Earth, and the entire universe puts a holy fear inside of me.

Having a holy fear is a positive thing. It keeps my relationship with God in perspective and balanced. "The fear of the Lord is the beginning of wisdom" (Psalm 111:10).

Read Hebrews 4:7 again. We are warned to listen to the Holy Spirit's voice and not to harden our hearts. To keep our hearts from being hardened, we must confess our sins, repent and turn away from them. Everything hidden in that secret place of our heart will be exposed, and nothing will remain hidden from God's sight. We will all give an account of our disobedience; no one will be excused. Money cannot buy our way out of trouble with God. He cannot be bought, because He created everything, and it all belongs to Him.

Hebrews 4:12 is powerful; it states, "The word of God is living and active and penetrates so deep that it divides our soul and spirit." That verse is so deep that we can't wrap our minds around the concept. Only God can explain how this is possible. God is the only person that can judge our thoughts and attitudes. We already have read that no human can see or judge our spiritual heart or know our thoughts. We must confess our sin and surrender to God's authority, regardless of the sacrifice or cost. Nothing that we suffer in this earthly life can compare to God's judgment. Yes, He is a loving God, and that is why He has to discipline His children: to save us from ourselves and to teach us. God's love is rich and much deeper than our human love, and His love is why He must hold us accountable.

The heart is deceptive; it can be filled with the desires of the flesh. When I refer to the flesh, I am referring to lust, greed, selfishness, jealousy, and yet more. The world teaches, "If it feels good, do it." That is deception and a lie. Who is the master of lies and deception? _____

In your Bible turn to Genesis, chapter 3, and read verses 1–19. Then read verse 13 again, and fill in the blanks below.

The woman said, "The _____ _____me, and I ate."

Satan was so deceptive that he had convinced Adam and Eve that the lie he was offering was good and true. He intentionally tricked them into believing that God did not really want them to be under his authority, due to his own selfishness. The Serpent made them doubt that God was protecting them from evil and death. Satan is still doing this today with each of us. Satan was so crafty with his words and twisted them into a believable lie for Adam and Eve. They gave in to the pressure of receiving pleasure for their own gain, without even thinking of the hurt and pain they would inflict on the most holy God, the one who provided everything for them, the one who gave them life! Are we giving in to the pressures of this world for our comfort and gain, still causing the same pain to our heavenly Father? Adam and Eve did not intentionally set out to rebel against God, they were deceived!

Sin was introduced into the world because two people hardened their hearts to the words and the warnings from our holy God. They disobeyed and were punished for their bad choice, sin. The tone was set for our world today. We now know what it means to sin and that we will be held accountable for our disobedience to God's authority.

In your Bible, read Genesis 3:14–19 again.

What was the punishment for the Serpent?

_____

_____

_____

_____

What was the punishment for Eve?

_____

_____

_____

_____

What was the punishment for Adam?

_____

_____

_____

_____

Are we still suffering the consequences for Adam and Eve's disobedience? Explain your answer.

_____

_____

This was Satan's ultimate plan. He was not only concerned with corrupting Adam and Eve; he used them to alter God's plan for mankind. He knew that if he could deceive them and lead them into sin, he would have access to the future generations. This is how he obtained access to us. We are still suffering the consequences of their sin, and the generations after us will also suffer the consequences of our sins. Our children, our grandchildren, and our great-grandchildren can and will be affected by the consequences of our poor choices and sins that we commit today, just as with Adam and Eve's . How many generations has that been?

God's plan is perfect, and He has a word of truth for the provision to defeat Satan.

Read Genesis 3:19 again. Now read John 3:16–17. How does Jesus impact Genesis 3:19?

Satan's agenda has not changed. He still wants to confuse, conquer, steal, kill, and destroy all of what God has created. "The thief comes only to steal and kill and destroy" (John 10:10).

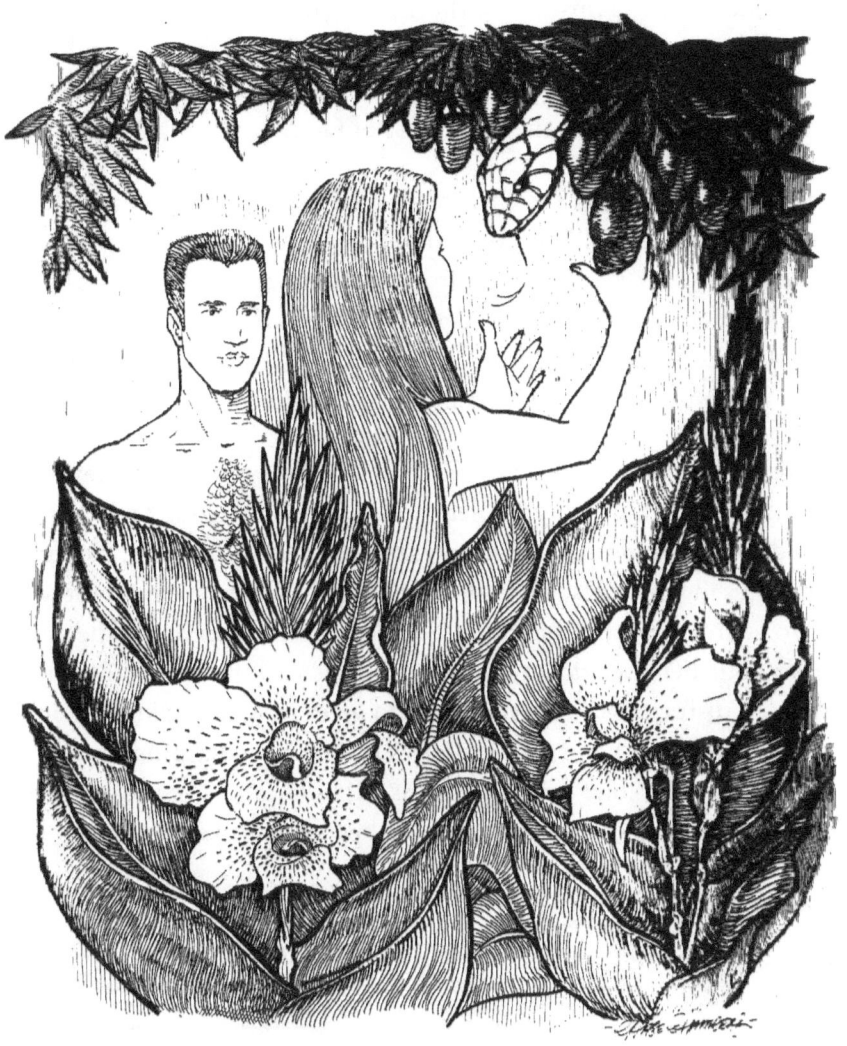

The serpent's deceit leads to the fall of Adam and Eve.

This is why God has provided the armor for this battle. The Enemy is still attempting to undermine God and His perfect plan. We must not forget that God warns that "our struggle is not against flesh and blood, but against the rulers, against the authorities, against the powers of the dark world and against the spiritual world and against the forces of evil in the heavenly realms." In Ephesians 6, we are warned to be prepared at all times by purposely "putting on the full armor of God."

Our heavenly Father is the picture of a perfect, loving parent. He has already established a plan for each of us, as a provision to bring us out of our personal deserts and free us from the bondage of sin. His ultimate goal is for each of us to have a testimony of His unfailing love, mercy, and grace. And to give us all an inheritance of eternal life, which will ultimately glorify and bring honor to Himself!

"Do not be anxious about anything but in everything, by prayer and petition, with thanksgiving, present your requests to God. And the peace of God, which transcends all understanding will guard your heart and your minds in Christ Jesus" (Philippians 4:6–7). It's very important to ask God to guard our hearts and minds, because sin starts in both. The second you let your defenses down and you're in a weak moment, the Enemy will try to distract and deceive you. God gives us warning in the book of Ephesians to be alert and arm ourselves for protection against the Devil's schemes. In the Bible, read Ephesians 6:10–17, and list the individual pieces of armor and their purpose in the spaces provided.

1. Ephesians 6:14

_____

_____

_____

2. Ephesians 6:15

_____

_____

_____

3. Ephesians 6:16

_____

_____

_____

4. Ephesians 6:17

_____

_____

_____

According to verse 12, who are we struggling with?

_____

_____

_____

_____

Read Ephesians 6:18 How are we to pray? _____

Why do you think we are warned to be alert? Remember the warning in Ephesians 6:12?

_____

_____

_____

_____

In verses 11 and 13, you are instructed to put on the full armor of God, to purposely put on the individual pieces, to clothe yourself with them. How do we stand firm with the belt of truth buckled around our waist, with the breastplate of righteousness in place? The breastplate of righteousness gives you a picture of a protective covering that will protect your spiritual heart.

The belt and the breastplate are ancient defensive gear that were worn for preparation for battle and for protection against the enemy. We must know and believe by faith that the truth is presented in God's Word. We must also know the person who is truth, Jesus Christ. Through our relationship with Him, and believing that we were made righteous by the shedding of His blood upon the cross, we have been set apart and are protected from the Enemy.

How do we take up the shield of faith? A soldier would hold his shield up in front of himself or herself to protect from bodily injury. While a physical shield protects us physically, faith protects us spiritually, even in the midst of difficult times.

Satan is always at work trying to cast doubt and fear into our everyday lives. These are his fiery darts to keep us distracted from God and the truth. Our defense is believing and asking by faith for God to take control. God is purposely working out every situation for our good and for His glory. "And we know that in all things, God works for the good of those who love Him, who have been called according to His purpose" (Romans 8:28).

Our shields are only as strong as our faith. If our faith is weak, our shields will not protect us. We must totally trust and believe that God's Word is our only absolute defense. His Word was truth thousands of years ago, and it is the same truth today. It has not changed, and God has not changed.

What is the helmet of salvation? A Roman soldier's helmet protected his head from injury while in battle. Salvation is received when we accept Jesus Christ as our personal Lord and Savior. Without the helmet of salvation, we would be unprotected and overcome with worry, doubt, and fear. Our thoughts would keep us in bondage, and we would become captives of this world. Remember Romans 12:2: "transformed by the renewing of your mind."

What is the sword of the spirit? We all know that a soldier's sword was his main means of attack. The sword is the only weapon that Paul listed as able to bring death to the Enemy. Read Hebrews 4:12. The word of God is living and powerful, and sharper than any two-edged sword, piercing even to the division of soul and spirit, and joints and marrow. The word of God can discern the thoughts and intent of the heart.

The sword of the living God is the all-powerful living Word of God. It is our only defensive weapon that can disable and disarm Satan. Jesus is our example to follow. Read Matthew 4:1–11. In the spaces below write out the verses.

Matthew 4:4

_____

_____

_____

_____

_____

_____

Matthew 4:7

_____

_____

_____

_____

_____

_____

Matthew 4:10

_____

_____

_____

_____

_____

_____

To whom was Jesus speaking? _____

Was Jesus in a spiritual battle or a physical battle? _____
Explain your answer.

_____
_____
_____
_____
_____
_____
_____
_____
_____
_____
_____

Satan will try to use your hardships and your circumstances against you. He will attack when you are distracted, and he will attempt to deceive you. He knew Jesus was hungry after forty days and forty nights in the desert. Remember, Jesus was a man while living on earth, and He experienced hunger, discomfort, and pain just as we do. The Enemy tried to use Jesus' hunger to trick Him into using His power to prove Himself and to make Him unlike man. Satan failed at deceiving Jesus in verses 5, 6, 8, and 9 of Matthew 4. What did Jesus use as His defense against the Devil's schemes?

_____
_____
_____
_____
_____
_____
_____
_____

Read Matthew 4:11 again. Who won the battle? _____

God's perfect plan has included a way for all of His children to be equipped for Satan's attacks. "Pray also for me, that whenever I open my mouth, words may be given me so that I will fearlessly make known the mystery of the gospel" (Ephesians 6:19).

"All scripture is God breathed and is useful for teaching, rebuking, correcting and training in righteousness, so that the man of God may be thoroughly equipped for every good work" (2 Timothy 3:16–17).

We are to speak God's Word in total faith and without fear of it failing. We are to speak God's Word with authority because we were given the right to speak with authority when we accepted Jesus as our Savior. The mystery of the gospel will be made known to others by the result of our acts of faith and our obedience. Many mysteries of God's Word were made known to man by Jesus' response to trials and temptations. Jesus lived out the Word of God by spending time with the Father in prayer and petition; by doing this He was putting on His armor. That is the example we are to follow and are to learn by His perfect life. We are to study the character of Christ and pattern our lives after His, so others can learn more about Him by the way we live. Believe in the Lord Jesus Christ, and seek Him with all your heart. Remember always: Ask and Believe that Christ will always be there and has already provided the way by truth!

XI

OUR MOTIVE FOR PHYSICAL TRAINING

The intentional practice of discipline is a form of worship to God. Let's change our attitude about exercise. Instead of making it something we dread, let's make it a time of worship. Exercise is a sacrifice, and it requires effort. If we choose to give up fattening foods and make better choices in our diets, it's a sacrifice. It can be used as an offering to God. Prayerfully and purposely start changing your source of motivation by giving up control, and sacrifice your own pleasures.

A consistent practice of discipline will bring balance into your life. The balance will be another reflection of Christ's character. Never in the Scriptures does it insinuate that Jesus had a discipline or scheduling problem. He made time to pray, to rest, to eat, and time to disciple (teach) others about God. He never had an issue with authority, even when He stood before Pilate. Think about it: this was the son of God, and he had the power to stop His judgment.

He was obedient and under submission to God's authority first and then to Pilate. Jesus always had order and control of his prayer life, which enabled him to keep his emotions, actions, and motives under control. Prayer was the most valuable and most powerful tool that Jesus had available to complete His Great Commission.

His Great Commission was to show us God by example and to endure the crucifixion, to save mankind. Jesus' prayer life was his direct communication with His Father, and that is how He achieved so much in thirty-three years. Jesus completed His task, and we should pattern our lives after His. Our source of motivation to improve our physical bodies should not be for the world's acceptance, but to honor God. We should offer our bodies as a sacrifice to better serve Him. The world wants you to focus on the outside, but God wants you to focus on the inside.

If you honor Him by making sacrifices and start practicing discipline for Him, as a blessing, the outside will take care of itself.

Memorize 1 Corinthians 6:19–20: "Do you not know that your body is a temple of the Holy Spirit, who is in you, whom you have received from God? You are not your own; you were bought at a price. Therefore, honor God with your body."

Let's get started!

Ask God to bring everything that you have read and studied into your mind and heart; remember that we are continuing to renew our minds daily. Pray for God to make the connection of spiritual and physical training. Earlier in the study we discussed making everything eternal and to focus on bringing glory to God by everything we do, including exercise and nutrition. Develop an exercise class, and make it a time of worship and a sacrifice to bring glory to God, with the mind-set of 1 Corinthians 6:19–20: "Do you not know that your body is a temple of the Holy Spirit, who is in you, whom you have received from God? You are not your own; you are bought at a price. Therefore honor God with your body."

Don't dread your time of exercise; make it a time of thanksgiving, and praise God for your having the ability to exercise. Make a *choice* to practice *discipline*! Choose to practice three basic elements of balance, which are nutrition, exercise, and rest. Remember that we have to renew our minds in *all* things: the way we approach the table, choosing to move instead of sitting, and purposely setting a bedtime. These simple elements were put in place by God, and there are consequences of not applying these basic principles. If we overeat and make bad nutritional choices, we will suffer from health issues, including obesity. If we do not choose to move and exercise, our muscles will atrophy, which causes deterioration of our joints and the premature breakdown of our bodies. If we choose not to get enough sleep, our bodies will age and weaken a lot quicker. Sleep gives our cells time to reproduce, which will rejuvenate our bodies. A balance of the three will assist with weight loss due to us having more energy, which will result in burning more calories and fat. We make it so hard, but it really isn't. But, again, it takes *discipline*!

God will honor and bless our efforts if we make it all about *Him*, and not about pleasing the world and being controlled by or consumed with our appearance. Make your motives and intentions all about living a life that is totally pleasing to God. Share any concerns or struggles with your accountability partner, and ask for prayer. Hold each other accountable for the next forty days, and renew your mind daily. Change your attitudes, and intentionally plan your meals, schedule your exercise, and get your rest. Due to our lack of understanding of how much power we as believers of Jesus Christ have obtained by simply believing, we have limited ourselves by not using the power that we have inherited and which is promised to us by our heavenly Father. *Ask* God to give you the power to practice daily discipline and *believe* that your relationship with *Christ* can give you the strength to succeed and reach your goal. Remember Romans12:1–2, and apply it to your physical training. Also, Ask and Believe in Christ …

Colossians 1:10–12 "And pray this in order that you may live a life worthy of the Lord and may please Him in every way: bearing fruit in good work, growing in the knowledge of God, being strengthened with all power according to His glorious might so that you may have great endurance and patience, and joyfully giving thanks to the Father, who has qualified you to share in the inheritance of the saints in the kingdom of light."

Pray with your accountability partner, and ask God to empower you with His strength to practice the daily discipline and to give you the recall of His Word for instruction and direction. Pray also for endurance to continue to the process of renewing your mind and to be patient for the change to start from the inside out. Restoration is a process and a daily choice to be continued as a lifestyle. Ask with a pure motive, and believe that what you ask for will be given, by faith! "You do not have, because you do not ask God. When you ask, you do not receive, because you ask with wrong motives" (James 4:2–3).

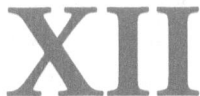

XII

Preparing Our Minds and Hearts for Physical Training

She sets about her work vigorously; her arms are strong for her tasks.

—Proverbs 31:17

Now that we have begun our spiritual training, know that it will not be completed until we die. The task that God has given each of us will require progressive spiritual and physical training. It is a huge and exhausting task. In Matthew 28:18–20, God gives us the Great Commission: Jesus said, "All authority in heaven and on earth had been given to me. Therefore, go and make disciples of all nations, baptizing them in the name of the Father and of the Son and of the Holy Spirit, and teaching them to obey everything I have commanded you. And surely I am with you always to the very end of the age."

I believe God didn't limit this commission to foreign nations. It includes our neighbors, coworkers, friends, enemies, relatives, and anyone that does not know Jesus. Wow, that's a lot of spiritual and physical work! God knew this would be a huge task, and he gave all the provisions to complete it.

Commission means that we have been authorized by God to perform certain duties or tasks. It will require having knowledge of his Word, and physical strength for the endurance to complete such a huge task.

A deep personal relationship with Jesus Christ is a requirement that cannot be compromised. To know Jesus is to know God and how much he truly loves us. (Read John 14:6–7.)

God's Word is our strengthening tool for spiritual matters, just as resistance weights are tools for strengthening our muscles in our physical bodies. His Word is always fresh and made like new. It never changes and is never failing. The world's view has changed and will continue to change. The Word of God had been the same for thousands of years. Remember, the Word of God is God breathed, and He will continue to supply new life into every word that is given to each of us at the exact time of need. Remember, 2 Timothy 3:16 says, "All the scripture is God breathed and useful for teaching, rebuking, correcting, and training in every need."

As we continue with our spiritual training, our foundation will grow stronger. We will begin to obtain more wisdom and develop more discipline. 1 Corinthians 3:9–11 says, "For we are God's fellow workers; you are God's field; God's building. By the grace God had given me, I laid a foundation as an expert builder, and someone else is building on it. But each one should be careful how he builds. For no one can lay any foundation other than the one already laid, which is Jesus Christ."

Continue to pray for God to expose anything in your heart that could cause you to have a "diseased heart." We talked about the results or symptoms from unresolved issues that might be buried deep in our hearts, things like unforgiveness, selfishness, lying, greed, hatred, bitterness, rebellion, pride, and jealousy. In other words, unconfessed sin without repentance.

This is a dangerous condition that could hinder your prayers from being heard by God. Your heart could be hardened toward God, and you could possibly start blaming Him for all your troubles. If this "diseased heart" goes untreated, you will develop a condition of "prayerlessness," and that cuts you off from God. If unresolved issues are kept inside and not addressed, they could lead to serious addictions (including to food and to overspending). We have the need to feel satisfied with *something*. Be satisfied with *Jesus*.

We all know that any addiction has serious consequences. Stop and pray for God to reveal anything suppressed or hidden in your heart that might keep you in denial or stuck in your personal desert. Read Ezekiel 36:26–27: "I will give you a new heart and put a new spirit in you; I will remove from you your heart of stone and give you a heart of flesh. And I will put my spirit in you."

Let us reflect back on what we have already discussed and studied about the character of Christ. Turn to Matthew 5:1-11, and pray over these Scriptures for understanding. These scriptures are so important for our spiritual training we will study them again later. Absorb and digest these teachings. The Beatitudes are teachings directly from Jesus. Internalize them to be renewed from the inside out. Read them and process them in your mind, but transfer your understanding into your heart for daily application.

Now, having this head knowledge of Jesus is not enough. We also have to have the heart knowledge to pattern our life after His example; therefore, change has to take place. Without the heart knowledge, which is given by the Holy Spirit, there is no desire for change. We have to choose to be no longer conformed to the pattern of this world, but to be transformed by the renewing of our minds (Romans 12:1–2). Choose to change from the inside out. It starts in your heart when you accept Jesus Christ as your personal Lord and Savior. Our hearts and attitudes should mirror the very heart of Christ.

Continue to pray with faith and without ceasing. Remember we are a restoration project not completed until we meet God. This process will require wisdom, guidance, and strength to develop the spiritual and physical discipline required to complete our task and to overcome any addiction or sin.

What does *discipline* mean? Webster's says it means "training that develops self-control and character: the result is of such ordaining orderly conduct; submission to authority and control." The word *discipline* derives from *disciple*. I find it interesting that these words interact so closely within the life of Jesus. God gives insight and warning as to how important discipline is, and that it should be applied in our daily lives. Do not confuse being disciplined with being compulsive. Discipline is being in control; being compulsive is being under the control of something, which can include overspending and overexercising. Proverbs 5:23 says, "_____will die for the lack of discipline, led astray by his or her own great folly." (put your name in the blank provided and make this verse personal). These are very direct and strong words given by God for our training and teaching. He knows how weak we are and how we are going to be tempted by the foolishness of this world. "For the wisdom of this world is foolishness in God's sight" (1 Corinthians 3:19).

God is a God of order, and He wants us to live a disciplined lifestyle. Our obedience to His instruction will reflect His image to a lost world. Our actions can speak louder than our words. To be a reflection of God to the world is impossible without total submission to God and His Word as the authority over our lives. By making bad choices due to the lack of submission and ignoring His valuable teachings, I have made my life harder than what God intended it to be. I just kept going deeper into that same old desert to chase after the foolishness of this world and try to make myself happy. I just needed to find rest and fulfillment with I had already been given. The lesson that God was trying to teach me was to find satisfaction right where I was, and that my joy had to come from inside out.

My motivation had to change 100 percent. I had to become more eternally motivated, not temporally motivated: in other words, live for Christ and not for self. I needed to be more concerned about God's opinion of me, and less concerned of people's opinions. The source of our motivation is what pleases God. Read Proverbs 16:2–3: "All a man's ways seem innocent to him, but motives are weighed by the Lord. Commit to the Lord whatever you do and your plans will succeed." Commit your physical training to the Lord, and make it all about Him.

We cannot play games with God; remember that He sees what is hidden in those secret places. He knows our every thought and the true motivation behind our actions. 1 Corinthians 4:5 says: "Therefore judge nothing before the appointed time; wait till the Lord comes. He will bring to light what is hidden in darkness and will expose the motives of men's hearts. At that time each will receive praise from God." I also believe that we will be judged and held accountable for our impure motives and our sinful actions. We are forgiven, but there are consequences to every one of our sins. Praise God, we will not receive what we deserve. If we know Jesus Christ as our Lord and Savior, we are covered by His blood. The Father will give us mercy, and by His grace we will not be condemned into hell.

Let's think about who or what controls you. Are you self-controlled and disciplined, or are you controlled by something, such as an addiction or destructive behavior, or are you just totally out of control? Ask God to reveal to you anything that you need to change about your life that is not pleasing to Him and anything that keeps you from being obedient. Pray with your accountability partner, and seek the truth for your life.

2 Timothy 1:7: "For God did not give us a spirit of timidity, but a spirit of power, of love, and self-discipline." Amen!

XIII

Physical A, B, Cs ... Amounts, Balance, and Choices

Continue to focus and to reflect on Romans 12:1–2; it is still about changes from within. Pray for the strength and endurance required to make permanent lifestyle changes. Ask your accountability partner to pray that your focus will be on renewing your mind in regard to better health, and not entirely on weight loss and your appearance.

"Don't you know that you yourselves are God's temple and that God's spirit lives in you?" (1 Corinthians 3:16). Let your focus be on keeping your body and life God-centered. "Since then, you have been raised with Christ, set your hearts on things above where Christ is seated at the right hand of God. Set your minds on things above, not on earthly things"(Colossians 3:1–2).

In your own words, write out your understanding of each of these verses.

1 Corinthians 3:16

_____

_____

_____

Colossians 3:1–2

_____

_____

_____

Remember, let's keep it simple as A, B, C ...

A...Amounts

Before each meal plan and make intentional choices of preparing nutritional foods and choose to eat smaller portions at each meal. Pray for your accountability partner and for yourself to have the strength and discipline to make the necessary lifestyle changes for renewing your minds regarding your health and your bodies. Practice and develop the discipline of eating one-half of the amounts of food that you would normally eat at each meal. Read Colossians 3:1–2 again. Approach the table with these verses written in your mind and heart. As an offering and as a sacrifice to God, give Him one-half of what's on your plate. If you are in a restaurant, ask for a takeout box when you order your meal. When your meal arrives, put one-half of the food from your plate into the box, and eat the amount that is left. Save the rest for another meal, or share it with your spouse or friend. Give it up in the name of the Lord!

"And whatever you do, whether in word or deed, do it all in the name of the Lord Jesus giving thanks to God the Father through Him" (Colossians 3:17).

Let the verses 1 Corinthians 3:16, Colossians 3:1-2, and Colossians 3:17 become your motive for making your lifestyle changes.

Eat smaller amounts at each meal, with healthy snacks in between each one. Document each meal in your notebook. Keeping a record of your food choices and the amounts will help you to stay disciplined and focused. If you get off track and do poorly for a day, forgive yourself, share your mistake with your accountability partner, pray, and start again. Don't quit and don't give up.

Read the Scriptures written below; feed upon them and be filled and satisfied.

John 6:26–27:.Jesus said, "I tell you the truth, you are looking for me, not because you saw miraculous signs but because you ate the loaves and had your fill. Do not work for food that spoils, but for food that endures to eternal life, which the Son of Man will give you. On him God the Father has placed his seal of approval."

John 6:35: "I am the bread of life. He who comes to me will never go hungry and he who believes in me will never be thirsty."

Be filled with something other than food; focus on filling that empty spot in your heart, rather than on the false emptiness in your stomach. Don't be misguided and feed on comfort food that is only a temporary fix. "Let them give thanks to the Lord for His unfailing love and His wonderful deeds for men, for He satisfies the thirsty and fills the hungry with good things" (Psalm 107:8–9).

Does being overweight and the guilt of overeating keep you in captivity? Could this be your personal desert? "I am the Lord your God, who brought you out of Egypt [captivity]. Open your mouth and I will fill it" (Psalm 81:10).

We should eat when we are truly experiencing physical hunger and our bodies are in need of fuel to function. Remember to make wise choices and eat smaller amounts. We should not eat due to stress or discontentment; this is "emotional eating. Our emotions can give us a craving for comfort foods, which are usually our unhealthy junk foods. They are loaded with lots of empty fat calories that will give us a temporary sense of satisfaction. If we habitually continue in the cycle of emotional eating, we will end up obese, unhealthy, and depressed from guilt. When this false hunger occurs, fill up with spiritual food by turning to God in prayer, feed upon the Scriptures, or go on a prayer walk. Break the habitual cycle; get out of that desert. Go to Jesus and be filled.

B...Balance

Who has measured the waters in the hollow of his hand, or with the breadth of his hand marked off the heavens? Who has held the dust of the earth in a basket, or weighed the mountains on the scales and the hills in a balance?

—Isaiah 40:12

What is balance, and why do we need it? Balance is having equilibrium in the body, which means having harmonious proportions of weight distributed evenly throughout the body. We need it to be able to walk or to sit without support. Without physical balance we stagger, and sometimes we have to have a crutch. Without physical balance we eventually fall down.

That is a picture of what it's like to be off balance spiritually. God uses His physical creation to give us a clear understanding of what He wants us to truly to know about our need for Him and His truth. Balance is also required for our spiritual health; it's achieved by reading God's Word, by prayer and worship. Without it we stagger off track and wander in our own personal deserts, we possibly turn to things of the world for a crutch, and we eventually spiritually fall down.

Balance, spiritual and physical, is achieved by practicing discipline and obedience. Discipline yourself to achieve balance in the amounts of your daily nutritional intake, your daily exercise, and your daily rest. These three components have to balance for better health. God was very creative when he designed the human body with the intention for our bodies to be functional and maintainable until age overcomes them.

When I was studying physical therapy, I had the opportunity to see and study a human cadaver at the University of North Carolina. It was amazing to see the human body without flesh, and how intentional God was with

His design. Each part had a specific function, but for total function all parts works together. Humans will never design anything that will ever compare to God's creation of the human body. No wonder He modeled the church after it, because its function and purpose are so unique. Every single cell, bone, joint, muscle, and internal organ has a specific purpose. That tells me that He takes pride in our bodies, His creations.

This stands to reason, because He created us in His image. Genesis 1:27 says, "So God created man in His own image, in the image of God He created him; male and female He created them." Our bodies will not last forever—that's part of God's altered plan—but we can take care of them and try to preserve our precious gift of good health, being good stewards of all things. Remember, we have a Great Commission to live out until the end of our lives.

God referred to hunger and thirst throughout the Bible, which implies that He knew how important the two would be to humans. The Last Supper was a picture of the importance of gathering around the table, and Jesus chose to sit and eat with His disciples. He chose to use bread in reference to His body, and wine in reference to His blood. How significant is this? I say very, because Jesus chose it, did it, and said it; and thousands of years later it is still used in our belief and faith to remind us of His sacrifice. Jesus was so in tune with holy God, His Father; and everything He said and did was significant. Let's look at the references to hunger and remember that hunger is what we experience as a warning that we need nourishment, fuel for the body, to live. If we go without food, our bodies will deteriorate. Eventually we weaken and die. God chose to use hunger to give us a picture of how we also need to desire spiritual nourishment, that without it we deteriorate, weaken, and eventually perish. Jesus refers to Himself as the Bread of Life.John 6:32–35 states: "Jesus said, "I tell you the truth, it is not Moses who has given you the bread from heaven, but it is my Father who gives you the true bread from heaven. For the bread of God is he who comes down from heaven and gives life to the world. "Sir", they said, "from now on give us this bread." Then Jesus declared, "I am the bread of life. He who comes to me will never go hungry, and will never be thirsty." Psalm 107:8 says, "Let them give thanks to the Lord for His unfailing love and His wonderful deeds for men, for he satisfies the thirsty and fills the hungry with good things." Those good things are love, joy, peace, patience, kindness, goodness, faithfulness, gentleness, and self-control. You will be filled with everything needed to live a life pleasing to God, which will also enable you to develop the character of Christ.

The Lord's Supper gives us such a picture of what Jesus' focus was on even as He faced death. Read Matthew 26:17–30, and ask for the understanding of the hidden truths with your heart. In the spaces provided write out your understanding and significance of Matthew 26:17–30.

_____
_____
_____
_____
_____
_____
_____
_____
_____
_____
_____
_____
_____
_____
_____
_____
_____
_____
_____
_____
_____
_____
_____
_____

The disciples asked Jesus where should they prepare the Passover meal, and He replied, "Go into the city to a certain man and tell him, the Teacher says: "My appointed time is near. I am going to celebrate the Passover with my disciples at your house." His last meal was a celebration of His life, death, and resurrection. His conversations around the table were about His betrayal, and He was making provision for all seated there, and also for us. "While they were eating Jesus took bread, gave thanks and broke it, and gave it to his disciples, saying, 'Take and eat; this is my body.' Then taking the cup, gave thanks and offered it to them saying, 'Drink from it, all of you. This is my blood of the covenant, which is poured out for many for the forgiveness of sins'" (Matthew 26:26–28). God gives us a correlation of the spiritual and physical needs of food and drink. Jesus intentionally gives us a picture of the needs of what is good and pleasing for the soul and body. God gives us the options to choose good nourishments or bad. Both have consequences and we know which are good and which are bad.

Pray for God to give you wisdom and insight to develop balance. Commit to reading the Word of God, pray to and worship Him daily. Ask Him for help to assist with developing balance in the physical also. Start with discipline and obedience, and decide to make better choices. Use the suggestions written below to help you make changes to your daily nutrition; be intentional and *choose* to apply them at each meal. *Plan*!

Nutrition

God gave us the sense of taste to experience pleasure in our food and drink. He also relates the sense of taste to Himself, to give an understanding of how He can satisfy a craving in our heart and soul.

Psalm 34:8 says, "Taste and see that the Lord is good; blessed is the man who takes refuge in Him." 1 Peter 2:2–3 instructs, "Like newborn babies, crave pure spiritual milk, so that by it you may grow up in your salvation, now that you have tasted that the Lord is good." God also speaks of us being "filled" and "satisfied," which can also relate to our appetites. Can you remember the last big meal that you had, and that feeling of being content, your cravings completely satisfied? God has given us another correlation of spiritual satisfaction and physical satisfaction. I believe He used the physical and spiritual connection to give us a clear and better understanding of His Word. Jesus was so intentional with His daily life and teachings.

Isaiah 55:1–3: "Come, all you who are thirsty, come to the waters; and you who have no money, come, buy and eat! Come, buy wine and milk without money and without cost. Why spend money on what is not bread, and your labor on what does not satisfy? Listen, listen to me, and eat what is good, and your soul will delight in the richest of fare. Give ear and come to me." We can renew our thoughts and our minds and go to Him and be filled. Our cravings will change to wanting more of God's spiritual nourishment, and wanting less of the world's physical nourishment. His Word promises that we will be completely satisfied!!

Educate yourself in the nutritional values of the different food groups.

Making positive nutritional changes can result in lowering your blood pressure, prevent or improve diabetic conditions and result with significant weight loss.

Meals should be prepared with the mind-set of making them high in nutrients and low in fats and carbohydrates.

Increase your intake of whole grains, and eliminate wheat products.

Increase your intake of soy products, and decrease your dairy products.

Increase your intake of fruits and vegetables.

Prepare and cook foods with olive oil, because it contains the "good fats."

Increase your use of herbs, spices, lemons, and limes to flavor your foods.

Decrease your salt intake.

Increase your intake of lean chicken (without skin) and fish (baked, broiled, or grilled, not fried). Decrease your intake of red meat; it's harder to digest.

Increase your intake of unsalted nuts and dried beans (cook your beans with olive oil).

Increase your use of honey and other natural sweeteners; decrease your use of cane sugar and artificial sweeteners.

Read your labels before you purchase packaged food. Remember, the first three ingredients listed are usually the main ones. Look for organic or all-natural foods without preservatives.

Drink water! Eight 8-ounce glasses a day is recommended for good cell production and organ function. Add fresh lemon juice as a natural diuretic for less water retention.

Educate yourself and know what you are eating. Don't eat it just because it tastes good. We can be easily deceived if we aren't careful. Fill up with something other than food. Our cravings are most often not from stomach hunger. Often we might be trying to fill that empty spot in our hearts. Don't be misguided and feed on comfort food that will provide only a temporary fix. The Enemy will continue to put temptations before us to keep us stuck in that same old desert, to keep us from making changes that might be of eternal or physical value.

I find it very interesting that the very first sin introduced to the world was temptation in the form of a food, the forbidden fruit. It is pleasing to the eye and good to the taste. I believe there is a hidden warning here about temptation of comfort food for fulfillment. God specifically commanded Adam, "You are free to eat from any tree in the garden; but you must not eat from the tree of knowledge of good and evil. For when you eat of it you will surely die" (Genesis 2:16–17). Adam and Eve thought they were going to be filled and satisfied by eating that unhealthy piece of fruit, and for a moment they probably were. Don't we still do that today?

At that time the fruit was forbidden and not good for people. Today there are many foods that are not forbidden, but if we choose to eat foods that are unhealthy for emotional fulfillment, we will create an unhealthy relationship with food. The cycle of unhealthy emotional eating will begin, and there will be consequences. Your health and bodily functions will suffer.

Most aspects of our daily lives are based on relationships, with a person, money, or even food. Our relationships are either healthy or unhealthy. How we develop and nurture our relationships is our responsibility; whether they are good or bad is determined by our choices and motives. If we are unbalanced spiritually and physically, we'll most likely make the wrong choices, with the results of unhealthy and painful consequences.

Pray with your accountability partner to develop balance in your lives, so you can experience better health and live by obedience to God's plan. God has a plan and a purpose for your life and for your future generations. His plan for each of us comes directly from His own heart, and that makes it perfect and eternal. His plan will be revealed to all the generations by the way we choose to live out our lives. If we are obedient and balanced, it will teach them by example, even with healthy eating and exercise habits. "But the plans of the Lord stand firm forever, the purposes of his heart through all generations" (Psalm 33:11).

Exercise

Pray before you start any exercise program; examine your motivations. Do a reality check list. Ask yourself these basic questions.

1. Why am I interested in choosing to exercise and to eat healthier? Is it totally for weight loss, for appearance and the world's acceptance? Is it to improve my health and to honor God? (1 Corinthians 6:19–20)

2. Are my choices of change in diet and exercise going to be doable and lasting?

3. Will I be able to maintain my choices as I age?

Be realistic; don't look for a quick fix. Pray about lifestyle changes that will require a lifetime of discipline. One of the worst things that you could do to your body is to have a pattern of starting and stopping with good nutrition and exercise. It is not good for your muscles and organs. It keeps your body in an unbalanced cycle. Your body will not be able to consistently function at its best level. You will not feel good, and your body will eventually break down.

Remember, the exercise and diet that you choose will have to be continued to maintain your weight and to keep your body at it's most functional state. Make it doable and maintainable for a lifetime. Don't look for a quick fix!

Talk with your physician before starting any exercise program or making drastic changes in your diet, especially if you have preexisting health problems.

Transform your exercise into a time of worship and praise. You choose to make this possible by the constant renewing of your mind, as in Romans 12:1–2.

Health Benefits of Exercise

Regular exercise can help protect you from heart disease and stroke, high blood pressure, non-insulin-dependent diabetes, obesity, back pain, and osteoporosis, and can improve your mood and help you to better manage stress.

For the greatest overall health benefits, experts recommend that you do twenty to thirty minutes of aerobic activity three or more times a week, and some type of muscle-strengthening activity and stretching at least twice a week. However, if you are unable to do this level of activity, you can gain substantial health benefits by accumulating thirty minutes or more of moderate-intensity physical activity a day, at least five times a week.

If you have been inactive for a while, you may want to start with less strenuous activities, such as walking or swimming at a comfortable pace. Beginning at a slow pace will allow you to become physically fit without straining your body. Once you are in better shape, you can gradually do more strenuous activity.

How Physical Activity Impacts Health

Regular physical activity that is performed on most days of the week reduces the risk of developing or dying from some of the leading causes of illness and death in the United States.

Reduces the risk of dying prematurely.

❖

Reduces the risk of dying prematurely from heart disease.

❖

Reduces the risk of developing diabetes.

❖

Reduces the risk of developing high blood pressure.

❖

Helps reduce blood pressure in people who already have high blood pressure.

❖

Reduces the risk of developing colon cancer.

❖

Reduces feelings of depression and anxiety.

❖

Helps control weight.

❖

Helps build and maintain healthy bones, muscles, and joints.

❖

Helps older adults become stronger and better able to move without falling.

❖

Promotes psychological well-being.

Specific Health Benefits of Exercise

Physical effects

Daily physical activity can help prevent *heart disease and stroke* by strengthening your heart muscle, lowering your blood pressure, raising your high-density lipoprotein (HDL, or good cholesterol) levels and lowering low-density lipoprotein (LDL, or bad cholesterol) levels , improving blood flow, and increasing your heart's working capacity.

Regular physical activity can reduce blood pressure in those with *high blood pressure* levels. Physical activity can also reduce body fatness, which is associated with high blood pressure.

By reducing body fatness, physical activity can help to prevent and control this type of *non-insulin-dependent diabetes.*

Physical activity helps to reduce body fat by building or preserving muscle mass and improving the body's ability to use calories. When physical activity is combined with proper nutrition, it can help control weight and prevent *obesity*, a major risk factor for many diseases.

By increasing muscle strength and endurance, improving flexibility and posture, regular exercise helps to prevent *back pain.*

Regular weight-bearing exercise promotes bone formation and may prevent or slow down the process of *bone loss.*

Psychological effects.

Regular physical activity can improve your mood and the way you feel about yourself. Researchers also have found that exercise is likely to reduce depression and anxiety and help you better manage stress.

We know that exercise has positive effects on the brain. Researchers at Duke University demonstrated several years ago that exercise can be an effective antidepressant. Other research has shown that exercise can improve the brain functioning of the elderly, and may even protect against dementia. How does exercise improve mental health?

One theory for some of the benefits of exercise is that exercise triggers the production of endorphins. These natural opiates are chemically similar to morphine. They may be produced as natural pain-relievers in response to the shock that the body receives in exercise. Researchers are beginning to question whether these substances improve mood. Studies show that endorphins do not cross the blood/brain barrier easily. Their ability to relieve pain probably occurs at the level of the spinal cord, leaving some other mechanism responsible for the mental health effects of exercise.

Recent studies have found that exercise boosts activity in the brain's frontal lobes. We don't really know how or why this occurs. Animal studies have found that exercise increases levels of serotonin, dopamine, and norepinephrine. These neurotransmitters have been associated with elevated mood, and it is thought that antidepressant medications like Prozac also work by boosting these chemicals.

Exercise has also been found to increase levels of brain-derived neurotropic factor (BDNF). This substance is thought to improve mood, and it may play a role in the beneficial effects of exercise. BDNF's primary role seems to be to help brain cells survive longer, so this may also explain some of the beneficial effects of exercise on dementia.

The bottom line is that most of us feel good after exercise, and it's probably not from endorphins. Physical exercise is good for our mental health and for our brains. Someday we will understand it all better—but we can start exercising *today*.

Millions of Americans suffer from illnesses that can be prevented or improved through regular physical activity.

13.5 million people have coronary heart disease.

1.5 million people suffer from a heart attack in a given year.

8 million people have adult-onset (non-insulin-dependent) diabetes.

95,000 people are newly diagnosed with colon cancer each year.

250,000 people suffer from a hip fracture each year.

50 million people have high blood pressure.

Over 60 million people (a third of the population) are overweight.

(Sources: John Briley, "Feel Good after a Workout? Well, Good for You," *Washington Post*, April 25, 2006; James A. Blumenthal, et al., "Effects of Exercise Training on Older Patients with Major Depression," *Archives of Internal Medicine*, October 25, 1999; Michael Babyak et al., "Exercise Treatment for Major Depression: Maintenance of Therapeutic Benefit at 10 Months, " *Psychosomatic Medicine*, September/October 2000.)

Muscle inflexibility can restrict the back's ability to move, rotate, and bend.

Weak stomach muscles can increase the strain on the back and can cause an abnormal tilt of the pelvis.

Weak back muscles may increase the load on the spine and the risk for disc compression.

Obesity puts more weight on the spine and increases pressure on the vertebrae

and discs. Studies report only a weak association between obesity and lower back pain, however.

Benefits for Chronic Back Pain

People with sudden and severe back pain should not exercise. Exercise plays a very beneficial role in chronic back pain, however. In one study, for example, patients with back pain lasting for an average of eighteen months were assigned eight, one-hour exercise sessions over four weeks. They showed greater improvement in nearly every area, including reduced pain and increased capacity, compared to patients who did not exercise.

Exercise should be considered as part of a broader program to return to normal home, work, and social activities. In this way, the positive benefits of exercise not only affect strength and flexibility but also alter and improve patient attitudes toward disability and pain.

Repetition is the key to increasing flexibility, building endurance, and strengthening the specific muscles needed to support the spine for improving our posture. Some exercise programs used for prevention or treatment of chronic low back pain include the following.

Low-impact aerobic exercises. Low-impact aerobic exercises, such as swimming, bicycling, and walking, can strengthen muscles in the abdomen and back without overstraining the back. Programs that use strengthening exercises during swimming may be particularly beneficial for many patients with back pain. In one study, for example, pregnant women who engaged in a water gymnastics program had less back pain and were able to continue working longer.

Lumbar extension strength training. Exercises called lumbar extension strength training are proving to be effective. Generally, these exercises attempt to strengthen the abdomen, improve lower back mobility, strength, and endurance, and enhance flexibility in the hip and hamstring muscles and tendons at the back of the thigh.

Yoga, t'ai chi, and chi kung. These exercises combine low-impact physical movements and meditation. They are based on principles of disciplining the mind to achieve a physical and mental balance and can be very helpful in preventing recurrences of lower back pain. In one study, Pilates, an exercise practice that uses yoga principles, was helpful in a woman with progressive and disabling severe lower back pain from early sclerosis. This approach deserves further research.

Flexibility exercises. Whether flexibility exercises alone offer any significant benefit is uncertain. One study suggested that any benefits derived from flexibility exercises are lost unless the exercise regimens are sustained.

Retraining deep muscles. Studies are finding a link between lower back pain and impaired motor control of deep muscles of the back and trunk. According to these studies, contraction exercises specifically designed to retrain these muscles may be effective for patients with both acute and chronic pain.

It is important for any person who has low back pain to have an exercise program guided by professionals who understand the limitations and special needs of back pain and who can address individual health conditions. One study indicated that patients who planned their own exercise did worse than those in physical therapy or doctor-directed programs. Improper or excessive exercise can also cause back pain.

Exercise's Effects on Bones and Muscles

Exercise is critical for strong muscles and bones. Muscle strength declines as people age, but studies report that when people exercise they are stronger and leaner than others in their age group.

Effects of Exercise on Osteoarthritis

Joints require motion to stay healthy. Long periods of inactivity cause the arthritic joint to stiffen and the adjoining tissue to atrophy. A moderate exercise program that includes low-impact aerobics and power and strength training has benefits for osteoarthritic patients, even if exercise does not slow the disease progression. Many patients who embark on an exercise program report less disability and pain and are better able to perform daily chores and remain independent than their inactive peers. Older patients and those with medical problems should always check with their doctor before embarking on an exercise program. The following are useful exercises for osteoarthritis patients.

Strengthening exercises builds muscle strength. Some experts encourage patients to emphasize strengthening leg muscles as a first treatment step, even before using pain relievers. They fear that patients who rely on painkilling drugs may overuse knees, which do not have muscle tissue sufficiently strong to protect the joints from further damage. Strengthening the thigh muscles is certainly protective to those who have not developed osteoarthritis.

Range-of-motion exercises increase the amount of movement in a joint and muscle. The best examples are yoga and t'ai chi, which focus on flexibility, balance, and proper breathing. In one 2001 study, older adults who practiced the gentle movement, breathing, and meditation exercises of t'ai chi for ten weeks reported less pain than their peers who did not learn the technique.

Low-impact aerobic workouts help stabilize and support the joints. Cycling and walking are beneficial, and swimming or exercising in water is highly recommended for people with arthritis. (Arthritic patients would avoid high-impact sports, such as jogging, tennis, and racquetball.)

Some researchers are now focusing on power training, which involves improving the muscles' ability to move more rapidly against resisting forces, such as gravity. For example, such training helps people to stand up or climb stairs more quickly. Muscle power declines more rapidly than muscle strength and may be particularly important in older people.

Exercise's Effect on Fractures and Falls

Exercise is very important for slowing the progression of osteoporosis, and extremely important for reducing the risk for falling, which causes fractures. Falls are one of the leading causes of death in people over age sixty-five. Exercise helps build balance and flexibility, which reduces the risk of falling. Specific exercises may be especially helpful for reducing the risk for fracture.

Weight-bearing exercises are very beneficial for bones in people of all ages, even older people. This approach applies tension to muscle and bone, and the body responds to this stress by increasing bone density, in young adults by as much as 2 to 8 percent a year. Careful weight training can also be very beneficial for elderly people, particularly women. In addition to improving bone density, weight-bearing exercise reduces the risk for fractures by improving muscle strength and balance, thus helping to prevent falls.

Regular brisk long walks improve bone density and mobility. In one 2002 study, for example, older women reduced their risk of hip fracture by over 40 percent working out for just four hours a week.

Exercises specifically targeted to strengthen the back can be beneficial in improving posture and may even reduce kyphosis (hunchback) in people with osteoporosis.

Low-impact exercises that improve balance and strength, particularly yoga and t'ai chi, have been found to decrease the risk of falling. In one study t'ai chi reduced the risk of by almost half.

Effect of Exercise on Back Pain

People who do not exercise regularly face an increased risk for lower back pain, especially during times when they suddenly embark on stressful unaccustomed activity, such as shoveling, digging, or moving heavy items. Although no definitive studies have been done to prove the relationship between lack of exercise and lower back pain, sedentary living is probably a primary non-medical culprit contributing to this condition.

Rest

Jesus said, "Come to me, all you who are weary and burdened, and I will give you rest. Take my yoke upon you and learn from me, for I am gentle and humble in heart, and you will find rest for your soul. For my yoke is easy and my burden is light." (Matthew 11:28–30).

There are two types of rest that humans require for good health. There is physical rest for our bodies to rejuvenate; approximately seven to eight hours a night is required. Every part of the body is affected: the brain, nervous system, immune system, hormones, emotions, heart, lungs, and the list goes on. It has also been proven that sleep deprivation can cause weight gain. The lack of sleep can sabotage any attempt to lose weight.

To live longer, keep our bodies strong and healthy, help our brains stay sharp and focused, improve our memory, and keep our emotions positive and balanced; we need to recognize the importance of physical rest. We must choose to get plenty of rest. Choose to set your bedtime, and discipline yourself to stick to it.

The other type of rest is finding peace in your soul. Have you ever had difficulty going to sleep, or have you ever awakened from sleep, tossing and turning due to worries and problems? The rest that I'm referring to is explained in Matthew 11:28–30. Read it again and ask for the understanding of this passage.

Jesus offers an invitation to come to Him because we are tired due to trying to solve our problems on our own. He offers His yoke. The definition of the word *yoke* is something that binds or unites; to join together. By uniting with Jesus, we learn from His example. He has a gentle spirit and a humble and forgiving heart. Jesus provides the way of freeing us from bondage, worry, and sin, and that gives us the ability to rest; we know that by simply believing in Him, we unite with Him and are then able to go to the Father. Our worries and fears are taken from us, and our burdens are made light. This gives the soul rest.

This rest comes from knowing and trusting all the promises of God. This rest comes from that spiritual foundation built from knowing and believing in Jesus Christ as your Lord and Savior. This rest is secured by embracing the Word of God and immersing yourself in it daily. This is the process of renewing your mind. Spiritual rest comes from living without fear and knowing that God has everything under control and that He has our best interests at heart. He already knew of every trial and heartache that we would ever face, even while we were still in our mother's wombs.

Read Psalm 139:15–16: "My frame was not hidden from you when I was made in the secret place. When I was woven together in the depths of the earth, your eyes saw my unformed body. All the days ordained for me were written in your book before one of them came to be" (Psalm 139:15–16).

God had provided the perfect rest, and it started with a little baby boy. This precious baby was born in a simple stable and had a manger for a bed. God intentionally allowed His Son, the King, to be born in a lowly stable to give us a clear picture of simplicity. He met the need of His child; the stable served the purpose and didn't have to be elaborate or a palace. The stable and the manger formed a humble and a precious setting for such a special and humble child to be born. This setting gave the world a clear picture of what we should embrace for our basic needs for our lives: *Simplicity*!

God provided an eternal rest by allowing that child to grow into a man to be our example of Himself. Jesus is our perfect picture of God, and He took on the sins of the world. He was killed because of His love for us, and His obedience to God cost Him his life. This complete rest is still available by His Spirit, because He overcame death. His Spirit, the Holy Spirit, is very much alive and continues to communicate the truths from our Father in heaven as we complete our earthly journey. God has provided a way for us to have spiritual rest. It comes from having the peace of Christ by knowing and believing that He has every problem and burden under His control.

John 16:33: I have told you these things, so that in me you may have peace. In this world you will have trouble. But take heart! I have overcome the world.

Colossians 3:15: Let the peace of Christ rule in your hearts, since as members of one body you were called to peace.

Philippians 4:6–7: Do not be anxious about anything but in everything, by prayer and petition, with thanksgiving, present your requests to God. And the peace of God, which transcends all understanding, will guard your hearts and your minds in Christ Jesus.

We must completely trust Him by faith and believe that He will work all things for good to bring glory to Himself and also to mature our faith. "And we know that in all things God works for the good of those who love Him, who have been called according to His purpose" (Romans 8:28).

Physical rest is made possible and is more enriched by having faith, believing the Word of God, and knowing Jesus Christ. We can have complete physical rest by being able to "sleep in heavenly peace." In other words, if it's well with our souls, we will have complete rest, both spiritual and physical.

C...Choices

I have to be reminded again and again that there are consequences to my choices, whether good or bad. I must pattern my life in a disciplined lifestyle to keep my focus on things above and not on the things of this world that will not last. I have to choose to keep my mind renewed daily, and always remember it's an ongoing process. Again, meditate on Romans 12:1–2.

Choose to offer your body as a living sacrifice, holy and pleasing to God; this is your act of worship. Choose not to conform any longer to the pattern of this world, but be transformed by the renewing of your mind (Romans 12:1–2).

How do we learn to make good choices? How do we get to the point of feeling satisfied and not feeling empty? We do so by having an understanding of what is truly of value and what will last. The truth is my most valuable possession. The truth reveals everything that is of eternal value and supplies all my needs. The truth is my resource of knowledge and understanding of Jesus Christ. The truth is revealed to me daily by the Holy Spirit. By seeking an understanding of the truth, I have developed a deeper relationship with Jesus, the Father, and the Holy Spirit. My greatest and the only reliable source of accountability should be the Trinity: the Father, Son, and the Holy Spirit, which are all supported by the truth! We have to grasp the need of this understanding to develop the ability and to have the power to make wise choices throughout life and be completely satisfied right where we are, regardless of the circumstance or situation, even in the midst of the most horrific storm!

"May the God of hope fill you with all joy and peace as you trust in Him, so that you may overflow with hope by the power of the Holy Spirit." Romans 15:13 By reading and understanding the Word of God and recognizing the value of its teachings, our minds will be filled with truth, and our hearts will be filled with the understanding of His love and His peace, which will bring us into His rest. This place of rest will keep us from being anxious or discontented, instead feeling completely satisfied. We can be transformed into the image of Christ, and we will require less to be completely happy and content with ourselves. To be filled up with Christ will decrease the need of being of the world and it's distractions. Staying focused on eternal things will enable us to make wise and positive choices, especially if they are based on and are accountable by the Word of God. Remember in the spiritual A,B,C we talked about having a strong foundation to strengthen us spiritually. This will enable us to complete our journey according to God's plan that He has already meticulously designed for each of us. Ephesians 1:11 says, "In Him we were also chosen, having been predestined according to the plan of Him who works out everything in conformity with the purpose of His will."

By loving Jesus with all of your heart, soul and mind, you will be *restored*! You will be satisfied, and your cravings will change. The end result will be having more discernment and the ability to make good, sound choices that are pleasing to God.

Galatians 5:22–24: But the fruit of the spirit is love, joy, peace, patience, kindness, goodness, faithfulness, gentleness, and self-control. Against such things there is no law. Those who belong to Christ Jesus have crucified the sinful nature with its passions and desires (cravings).

Psalm 107:9: For He satisfies the thirsty and fills the hungry with good things.

Psalm 81:10: I am the Lord your God, who brought you out of Egypt (your personal desert). Open your mouth and I will fill it.

Matthew 5:6: Blessed are those who hunger and thirst for righteousness, for they will be filled.

There will always be struggles and temptations in our lives. It's our response and our choices that will determine our consequences. Sometimes we create our own struggles by our poor judgment and because of our weakness. If we focus on our flesh and satisfying our temporal desires, we'll be just like Adam and Eve. Satan will always try to deceive us and keep us distracted from God's Word and attempt to lead us into the wilderness, or desert. He wants us to be isolated in our own personal desert and dysfunctional. Satan does not want us to change and make better choices, especially if others might be influenced or take notice. He does not want us to glorify God with our lives.

Pray daily for God's direction and for His leading, before making any choices. Ask yourself if the consequence or result will bring glory to God or shame? If you earnestly seek God's counsel and guidance, He will give you an answer according to your needs and not your wants. Your degree of obedience will be revealed as to how you accept God's answer. In other words, if God answers in His will and not yours, can you accept His judgment and know that it is best? He will help you with your choices, from the smallest to the largest. Make the choice today to stay focused on the character of Jesus Christ. Choose to pattern your life after His example.

Remember to keep it simple: A ... Ask   B ... Believe in C ... Christ

XIV

RESTORED

Restore me, Lord, make me whole.

Touch me, Lord, restore my soul.

Teach me, Lord, make me complete.

Allow this child to sit at Your feet.

O, Father, hear my cry!

Show me, God, how to simplify.

I've ignored the teachings from my childhood past,

but the worldly life did not last.

You allowed me to have my own way.

Forgive me, Lord, for I went astray.

I wandered into my desert of pain and despair,

but you, my God, were always there.

By prayer and love, you brought me here;

You, O God, removed my fear.

Father God, only you could find,

the ways and words to renew my mind.

You are still at work in me,

not complete until Your face I see.

Father, I must always ask and believe in Christ,

for You sent your Son as a sacrifice.

Your love, Your truth and ways I must share,

to teach my children that You've placed in my care.

I must teach Your Word and the stories of old.

They must be prepared; O God, they must be told.

Help me, Lord, to teach them well,

and then to their children they will also tell.

Continue, Lord, to make me whole.

Touch me, Lord, restore my soul.

Still teach me, Lord, make me complete.

Allow this child to sit at Your feet.

XV

CLOSING PRAYER

Dear heavenly Father,

I come to give You praise and to thank You for all that You have done for us. I recognize that You sacrificed Your only Son, Jesus Christ, to provide us with eternal life. Forgive us when we wander without Your direction; thank You for not leaving us in our personal deserts of pain and despair. We pray, Lord, that You will restore us by giving an understanding of Your Holy Word and showing how to apply it daily. Father, teach us how to renew our minds and start the process that will change us from the inside out. Please reveal and forgive us of any sin that we need to confess and repent of. Show us the secret places in our hearts where we have buried past pain and unforgiveness. Help us to forgive and heal our diseased hearts. Father, teach us to be satisfied and how to be filled. I pray that whoever reads this material will have a better understanding of your Son, Jesus Christ, and will develop a desire to have a deeper relationship with Him. God, I am interceding for those who are wandering without direction, and I *ask* that you show them the way out, I *believe* that you will never leave or forsake any of your children, and I know that a deep personal relationship with *Christ* is the answer. I pray that many will read the *truth* and be *restored*. Amen!

XVI

Leader's Guide

1. Plan a meeting for once a week. Arrive 15 minutes early to prepare for the session and be prepared. If this material is going to be used out of a group setting just modify the instructions and apply them accordingly, but try to follow the guidelines for the use of the written materials closely.

2. Begin and end each session with prayer.

3. The first 40 minutes of each session should be used for spiritual training. As an example: the first 5 minutes for prayer with the large group, 15 minutes for accountability partners to meet and discuss how they answered the questions or filled in the blanks and present prayer request, 20 minutes to discuss the material for the session in the large group. Remind everyone to record prayer requests in their notebooks. Be creative and let the Holy Spirit lead you. The exercise class should begin after each session of the spiritual training. The total time of combined sessions should be approximately 1 hour and 20 minutes. Try to keep your session time as scheduled.

4. Divide into groups of 2 to develop accountability teams. You may have a group larger than 2 if your total number is uneven.

5. Have the music and your exercise routine prepared. The exercise session should last approximately 40 minutes, 5 minutes of stretching, 30 minutes of strengthening/cardio and 5 minutes for cool down.

6. The assignment for the group should be given prior to the week of discussion, starting with session ONE at your fist meeting. Count the days to ensure you have your last meeting on or after the 40th day.

SESSION ONE: 1: Have a sign up sheet available , ask for their phone numbers in case a meeting has to be rescheduled (avoid rescheduling if possible except for emergencies because it sends a message of not being important or a priority). Use this sign up sheet as your prayer list. Pray for each name on the list daily. 2. Have scales available for each each person to weigh and have them to record their weight in their notebook, remind them not to weigh again until the end of the 40 day journey. 3. The first assignment to be completed before the next session is as follows: Read I. Focal Verse Romans 12:1–2, II."My Testimony", III. Mission Statement, IV. Suggestions for Success and Support V. Start With a Strong Foundation-"Steps To Receive Christ" and XI. Our Motive For Physical Training. Start your first exercise class and ask they do the exercises 2 more times during the week. Remind them to also schedule their time to walk with their accountability partner if possible.

SESSION TWO: VI. The Significance of the Number 40 Vll. Are We Any Different Than The Israelites, VIII. The Call, IX. The Ten Commandments and XII.Preparing Our Hearts For Physical Training

SESSION THREE: X. The Spiritual A,B,Cs...read ASK and XIII. Physical A,B,Cs read AMOUNTS . Remind each person to pray and meet with their accountability partner. Review Suggestions for success. Instruct the group to do their homework and focus on renewing their mind.

SESSION FOUR: X. The Spiritual A,B,Cs... read BELIEVE and in XIII. Physical A,B,Cs read BALANCE, Ask the group to discuss with their accountability partners.

SESSION FIVE: Assign the group to read The Spiritual A,B,C,s...read CHRIST and in Physical A,B,C s read CHOICES

SESSION SIX: Have the scales available for everyone to weigh because the 40 day journey should be completed. Positive results should be the blessings for the group if it has focused on the renewal of their mind, practiced obedience and applied the discipline of making better choices, spiritually and physically. Remember this is not a "quick fix" but it is the beginning of a lifetime commitment for spiritual and physical restoration. Discuss and briefly review each session and ask for testimonies of how God has worked for the past 40 days. After your exercise session read XIV. Poem;"RESTORED" and XV. The Closing Prayer.

It is recommended that you continue to meet weekly to pray, continue with the exercise class and for the accountability. The material can be recycled and used over and over. It can be used as a tool for refreshment and teaching. Encourage the ones that have finished the first 40 day journey to invite someone new to come and begin another journey with them. They would already be prepared and equipped to help someone else out of their personal desert by being their accountability partner. This is an ongoing process that can keep the ministry growing and can help with accountability for all involved. Remember the 40 day journey is only the beginning and the renewing of the mind is a lifetime commitment! Be a strong, enthusiastic and a prayerful leader. Be CONTAGIOUS!!!!!

LEADER'S GUIDE FOR EXERCISE INSTRUCTIONS

1. Read and follow each instruction carefully and practice to become confident and familiar with each exercise. Implement deep diaphragmatic breathing while performing each exercise.

2. Start each class with 5 minutes of stretching exercises, explain to the class the importance of preparing their muscles for the exercises to decrease soreness and to prepare them for the work-out. Perform each exercise slowly with an intentional, smooth stretching movement. Play slow relaxing music to set the tone for the stretching exercises and preparing the body for the exercises. Perform 10 repetitions of each of the exercises. Remind your class to deep breathe.

3. Instruct 5 minutes of cario exercise for the heart muscle and to increase the blood flow. March in place at a fast pace for 30 seconds and 30 seconds at a slow pace, alternating for a total of 5 minutes. You can

improvise the cardio segment with running, marching and dancing. Make it fun and use the appropriate music to encourage movement. The objective of this segment is to get the body moving !

4. Continue the class with 25 minutes of resistive exercises for the entire body's major muscle groups. Start with with 2-3 pound hand /ankle weights and gradually increase them as you progress with your exercises. Instruct your class to squeeze their hand weights to add resistance to the movement . When performing exercises to their legs, arms and spine always end the movement at the starting position and never jerk or strain. Instruct your class to perform the exercises slowly and to be intentional with the movement. Follow the sequence of the exercises provided in your leader's guide, start with 10-20 repetitions of each ex, the numbers will be determined by the age and physical condition of your group. You can modify the numbers of repetitions to meet the need of your class. Continue and encourage deep diaphragmatic breathing with all of the exercises.

5. End your class with 5 minutes of the stretching exercises that were performed at the beginning of the class. Perform them slowly with intentional, smooth stretching movement. Perform 10 repetitions of each exercise. Again use slow relaxing music for this segment and try to end your class relaxed and feeling good. Finish with 5 slow deep breaths!

6. Exercise prayer at the end of the session, ask for specific requests and pray for your group before ending the class.

*This is a simple guide to help get you started with an exercise class, you can be creative and progress your class as tolerated. Use the internet and credible exercise videos as other resources. Hold your class accountable and encourage the participants to hold each other accountable, also. * Discuss choosing a calorie level and introduce the chart that suggests the amount of calories according to your age and weight. Remind your class that the focus should be on improving health and being disciplined to enable them to serve our mighty God! Reflect and review the section of this study about having pure motives, Chapter XI. OUR MOTIVE for PHYSICAL TRAINING. Read Romans 12: 1-2 and 1 Corinthians 6:19-20.

FIND YOUR DAILY CALORIE LIMIT

WOMEN CURRENT WEIGHT	DAILY CALORIES	MEN CURRENT WEIGHT	DAILY CALORIES
125	1,500	150	1900
150	1,600	175	2,050
175	1,775	200	2,200
200	1,900	225	2,350
225	2,050	250	2,500

The chart above tells you how many net calories required each day to maintain your current weight. If you eat more, you will gain weight. If you eat less , you will loose weight. Find the numbers above that closely relates to you. To loose weight you must cut your calories and for faster weight loss cut at least 500 calories or more. A healthy weight loss is ½ to 2 pounds a week. It is healthier to loose the weight slowly and by loosing it slowly it will be easier to keep from gaining it back. You can loose weight by cutting calories or by burning them up by exercise. Remember it is the discipline and your motive for making healthier choices that will last a lifetime!

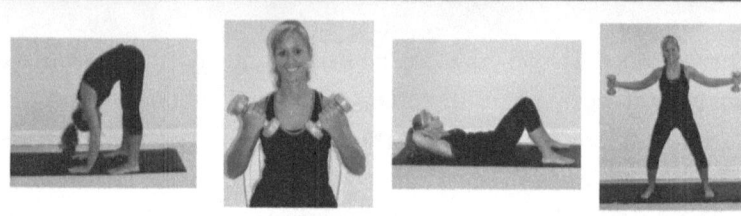

EXERCISES

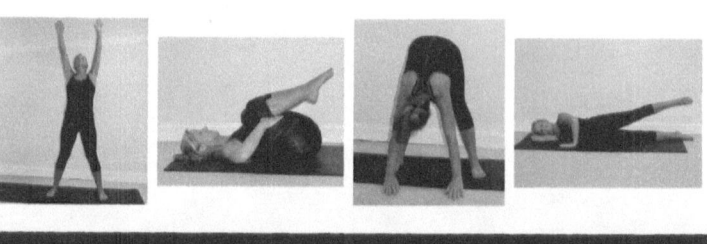

Romans 12:1 & 2

STRETCHING
EXERCISES

Sitting

Standing

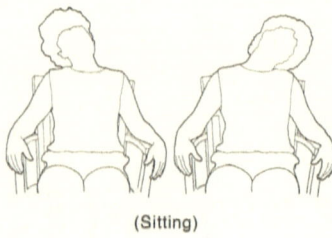

(Sitting)

Trunk and Neck - Lateral Neck Flexion

1. Tilt your head slowly towards your right shoulder, then your left shoulder, moving to the point of pain.

2. Do **not** rotate your head while tilting it or raise your shoulders.

3. Relax.

   Do _____ sets of _____ repetitions.

Special Instructions

Trunk and Neck - Lateral Neck Flexion /Extension

1. With you mouth closed, **slowly** lower you chin to your chest.

2. Bring your head back as far as possible so you can look up at the ceiling. Move gently, to the point of pain.

3. Relax.

   Do _____ sets of _____ repetitions.

Special Instructions

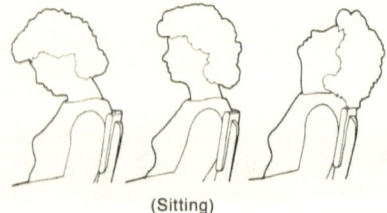

(Sitting)

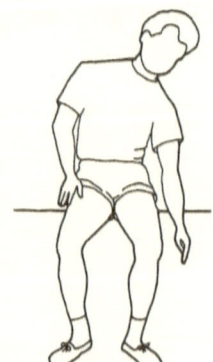

(Sitting)

Trunk and Neck - Lateral Trunk Flexion

1. Bend the trunk of your body to the left as far as possible.

2. Stretch your left hand towards the floor.

3. Hold for 5 seconds.

4. Return to starting position.

5. Repeat the exercise, this time bending to the right.

   Do _____ sets of _____ repetitions.

Special Instructions

Trunk and Neck - Forward Trunk Flexion

1. Bend forward and reach down to grasp the middle of your calves with both hands.

2. Hold for 5 seconds

3. Return to the starting position.
   Do _____ sets of _____ repetitions.

   Special Instructions

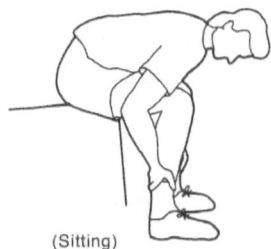

(Sitting)

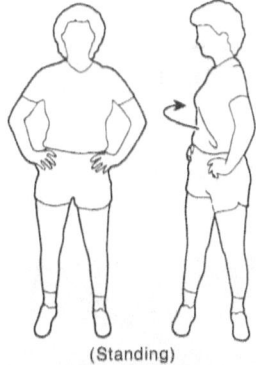

(Standing)

Trunk Range of Motion - Trunk Rotation

1. Stand upright with your arms on your hips and feet slightly apart.

2. Twist at the waist and look over your right shoulder.

3. Twist as far as you can, stopping at the point of pain.

4. Repeat on your left side.
   Repeat _____ times.

   Special Instructions

Trunk Range of Motion - Trunk Flexion / Extension

1. Stand upright with your arms relaxed at your sides and your feet slightly apart.

2. Bend forward and reach for your toes.

3. Stand back up and place your hands on the small of your back.

4. Lean backward and look toward the ceiling.
   Do _____ sets of _____ repetitions.

   Special Instructions

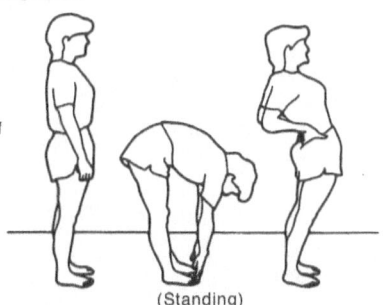

(Standing)

135

UPPER-BODY EXERCISES

Arms

Shoulders

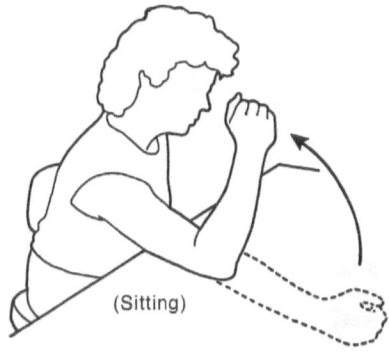

(Sitting)

Arms -- Elbow Flexion / Extension

1. Completely straighten your elbow

2. Bend your elbow

3. Return to the starting position.
       Repeat _____ times.

Special Instructions

Arms -- Shoulder Flexion

1. Start with your arms at your sides and the palms of your hands facing your body.

2. Bring your arms forward until your hands are level with your chin. Hold 5 seconds.

3. Bring your arms up until your hands are over your head.

4. Return slowly to the starting position.
       Repeat _____ times.

Special Instructions

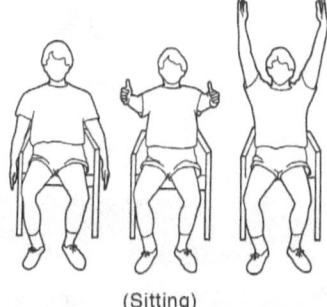

(Sitting)

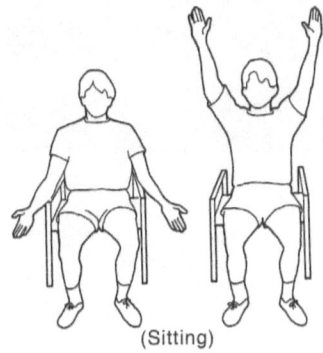

(Sitting)

Arms -- Abduction / Adduction

1. Start with your arms at your sides and the palms of your hands facing forward.

2. Lift your arms out to the sides and over your head. Keep your elbows straight.

3. Slowly lower your arms to the starting position.
       Repeat _____ times.

Special Instructions

137

LEG
EXERCISES

Sitting

Supine

Prone

Standing

Straight Leg Raises

- Tighten your thigh muscle with your knee fully straighted on the bed. As your thigh muscle tightens, lift you leg several inches off the bed. Hold for 5 to 10 seconds. Slowly lower.
  Repeat _____ times.

Special Instructions

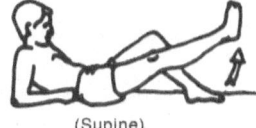

(Supine)

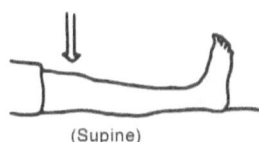

(Supine)

Quad Set

- Tighten your thigh muscle. Try to straighten your knee. Hold for 5 to 10 seconds. Relax
  Repeat _____ times.

Special Instructions

Hip Abduction

- Lie on your back. Keep you kneecaps pointed towards the ceiling throughout the exercise. Slowly move your involved leg out to the side of the bed as far as possible. Slowly return to starting position and relax. Repeat as instructed by your therapist.
  Repeat _____ times.

Special Instructions

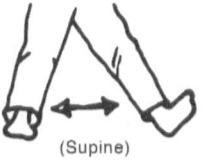

(Supine)

Ankle Pumps

- Slowly push your foot up and down. Do this exercise several times, as often as every 5 to 10 minutes. This exercise can begin immediately after surgery and continue until you are fully recovered.
  Repeat _____ times.

Special Instructions

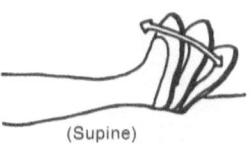

(Supine)

Hamstring Sets

1. Recline on your back, resting on your elbows.

2. Keep one leg straight, and bend the other to the height of about six inches.

3. Tighten the bent leg by digging down and back with the heel.

4. Hold for 5 seconds, then relax.
Repeat _____ times.

Special Instructions

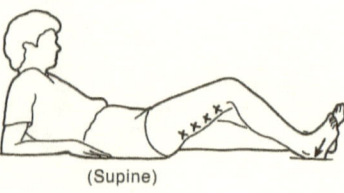

(Supine)

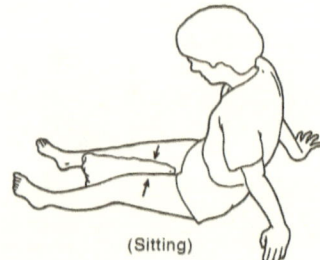

(Sitting)

Hip Adduction

1. Sit on a firm, flat surface with your hands behind you for support.

2. Straighten both legs and place a rolled towel between your knees.

3. Squeeze the towel roll between your legs for 5 seconds, then relax.
Repeat _____ times.

Special Instructions

Internal and External Rotation

1. Sit on a firm, flat surface with your hands behind you for support.

2. With your legs straight, turn your legs, from your hips to your feet, inward as far as possible.

3. Next, turn your legs, from your hips to your feet, outward as far as possible.

4. Be sure to turn your entire leg, not just the foot.
Repeat _____ times.

Special Instructions

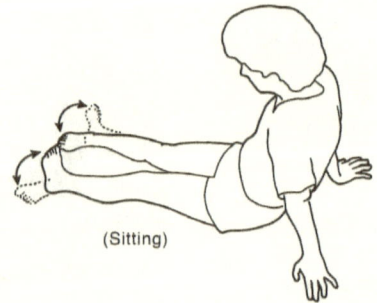

(Sitting)

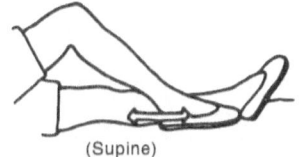

Heel Slides

- Slide your heel towards your buttocks, bending your knee on the bed. Do not let your knee roll inward.

  Repeat _____ times.

  Special Instructions

(Supine)

Gluteal Sets / Buttocks Contractions

Tighten your buttocks muscle. Hold 5 to 10 seconds.

Repeat _____ times.

Special Instructions

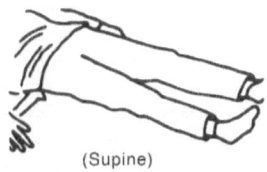

(Supine)

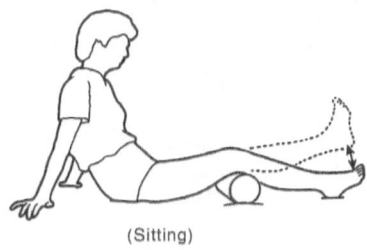

(Sitting)

Short Arc Quad

1. Sit on a firm, flat surface with hands behind you for support.

2. Place a rolled towel under one leg to bend it about 6 inches.

3. Raise the lower part of your leg until the knee is straight.

4. Hold for about 5 seconds, then relax.

   Repeat _____ times.

   Special Instructions

Hip Extension, Lying

1. Lie on your stomach with your arms folded under your head

2. Bend one knee so the foot points straight up.

3. Keeping your hips down flat, slowly lift the bent leg high enough to clear the other thigh.

4. Return to the starting position.

   Repeat _____ times.

   Special Instructions

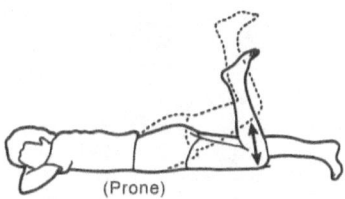

(Prone)

141

Long Arc Quad

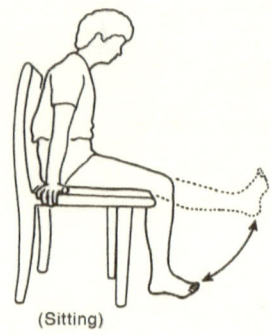

(Sitting)

1. Sit on a sturdy surface, high enough that your feet don't touch the floor.

2. Grip the sides of the surface for support.

3. Raise one foot until your knee is completely straight.

4. Slowly return to the starting position and relax.
   Repeat _____ times.

   Special Instructions

Legs - Hip Flexion

1. With your feet flat on the floor, lift your knee and raise your foot off the floor.

2. Hold this position for 5 seconds.

3. Put your foot down. Repeat the exercise with your other leg.
   Repeat _____ times.

   Special Instructions

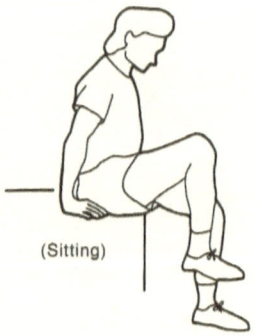

(Sitting)

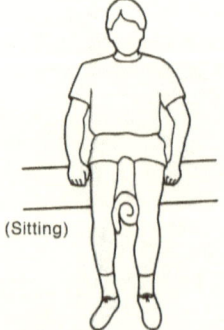

(Sitting)

Legs - Hip Adduction

1. Put a pillow between your knees and thighs

2. Squeeze the pillow tightly for 5 seconds. Relax.
   Repeat _____ times.

   Special Instructions

142

Mini - Squats

· Hold onto stable object (ie. chair or table) and slowly bend your knees. Keep both feet on the floor.
_____ times a day.
Repeat exercise _____ times. Hold position for___seconds.
_____
_____
_____

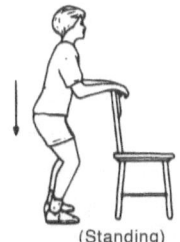

(Standing)

Hip / Knee Flexion

· Hold onto stable object (ie. chair or table) Stand with your feet slightly apart. Lift your right knee up to waist level. Return your foot to the floor. Repeat with your left leg.
Repeat _____ times.

Special Instructions

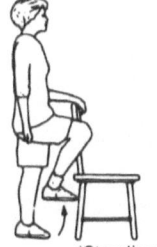

(Standing)

Toe / Heel Raises

· Hold onto stable object (ie. chair or table). Rise up on your toes and hold for ___ seconds. Rock back on your heel and hold for ___ seconds.
Repeat _____ times.

Special Instructions

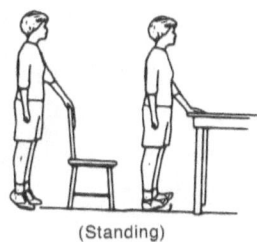

(Standing)

Hip Extensions

· Hold onto stable object (ie. chair or table), keeping your legs shoulder width apart and toes pointed forward. Slowly extend one leg back, keeping your knee straight. Do not lean forward. Repeat using other leg.
Repeat _____ times.

Special Instructions

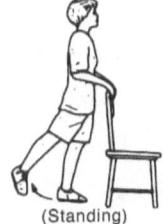

(Standing)

143

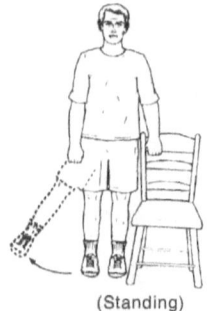

Hip Abduction

- Hold onto stable object (ie. chair or table) for balance. Move your leg out to the side then return to the starting position. Repeat exercise with your other leg.

  Repeat _____ times.

  Special Instructions

(Standing)

Sitting - Partial Sit to Stand

1. Sit on the edge of a firm surface and plant your feet.

2. Move your weight forward over your feet until your buttocks are just off the surface.

3. Lower yourself slowly until you are sitting upright again.

  Repeat _____ times.

  Special Instructions

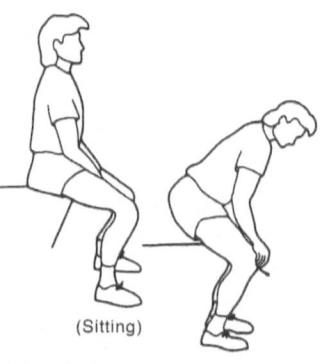

(Sitting)

Hamstring Curls

1. Lie on your stomach with your arms folded under your head, or stand near something that can be used for support.

2. Bend your knee, slowly bringing your heel up toward your buttocks.

3. Slowly return to the starting position and relax.

  Repeat _____ times.

  Special Instructions

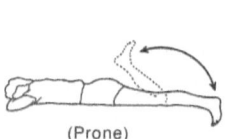

(Prone)

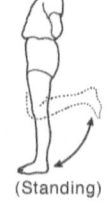

(Standing)

ABDOMINAL
&
BACK
EXERCISES

Supine

Hands & Knees

Prone

Partial Sit-Ups with Arms behind Neck

1. Lie on your back on a firm surface.

2. Lock your hands behind your neck. Curl your upper body forward until your shoulders clear the floor or bed.

3. Hold for 5 seconds. Relax.
   Repeat _____ times.

Special Instructions

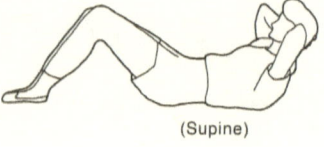

(Supine)

Bridging

1. Lie on your back on a flat surface.

2. Bend your hips and knees and plant your feet.

3. Raise your hips by pushing down evenly on both legs.

4. Hold for 5 seconds, then slowly lower your hips.
   Repeat _____ times.

Special Instructions

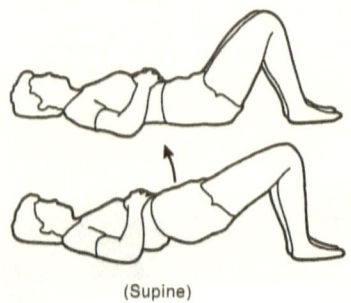

(Supine)

Cat Stretch

1. On a flat surface, get on your hands and knees. Put your hands under your shoulders and your knees under your hips.

2. Let your head hang down. Pull you stomach in and arch your back.

3. Hold for 5 seconds.

4. Slowly let your back sag and raise your head up.

5. Hold for 5 seconds. Relax.
   Repeat _____ times.

Special Instructions

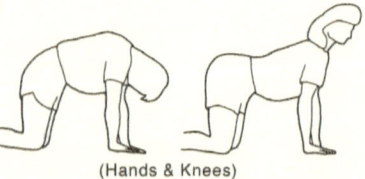

(Hands & Knees)

Quadruped Contralateral Arm and Leg Lift

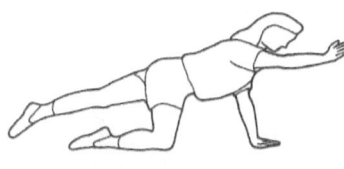

(Hand & Knees)

1. On a flat surface, get on your hands and knees. Put your hands directly under your shoulders and your knees under your hips.

2. Lift your right arm forward to shoulder level and you left leg to hip level. Keep your elbow and knee straight.

3. Hold for 5 seconds.

4. Repeat the exercise with your left arm and right leg.
   Repeat _____ times.

Special Instructions

Bilateral Shoulder Extension with Head and Shoulder Lift

1. Lie on a bed with a pillow under your body. Put a towel roll under your ankles or put your feet off the edge of the bed.

2. With your arms at your sides, lift both arms towards the ceiling, squeezing your shoulder blades together.

3. Now tilt you head and shoulders toward the ceiling, keeping your chest on the bed.

4. Hold for 5 seconds.
   Repeat _____ times.

Special Instructions

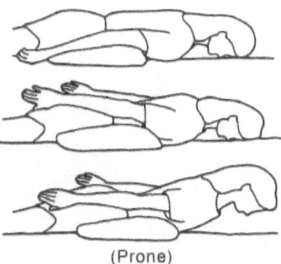

(Prone)

Prone Contralateral Arm and Leg Lift

1. Lie with you stomach on a pillow on a flat surface. (You can rest your head on a rolled up towel.)

2. Stretch your arms overhead and slightly to the sides of your head. Point your thumbs up.

3. Lift your right arm and left leg, keeping your knee straight and your hips flat.

4. Hold for 5 seconds.

5. Repeat the exercise with your left arm and right leg.
   Repeat _____ times.

Special Instructions

(Prone)

40 Day Journey

1	2	3	4	5	6	7
8	9	10	11	12	13	14
15	16	17	18	19	20	21
22	23	24	25	26	27	28
29	30	31	32	33	34	35
36	37	38	39	40		

Prayer Requests and Notes

Memorize: Therefore, I urge you, in view of God's mercy, to offer your bodies as a living sacrifices, holy and pleasing to God - this is your spiritual act of worship. Do not conform any longer to the pattern of this world, but be transformed by the renewing of your mind.   -Romans 12: 1-2

ABOUT THE AUTHOR

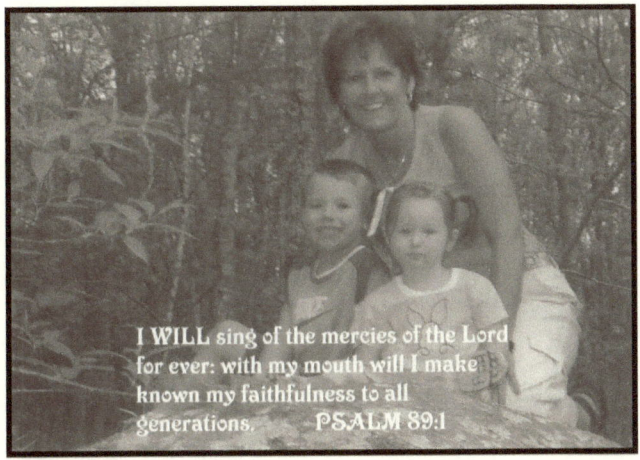

Donna is an ordinary person appointed by God to do an extraordinay thing. She shares her life experiences of being part of a dysfunctional family due to the devistating effects of alcohol abuse by her father in her formative years. The effects has caused her to be addicted to food and over spending to fill the emptiness in her heart. She shares her faith and how God's word has helped her overcome adversity. She has written of how God had a plan for her life and that He allowed her to wander into her personal deserts to teach her to be dependent upon the word of God and to seek a personal relationship with Jesus Christ, to be filled and satisfied. God had provided a godly mother and grandmother that taught her to ASK, BELIEVE in CHRIST. She wants to help others to renew their minds with TRUTH and start the process of physical and spiritual restoration.